STUDY GUIDE

for

Nutrition:
An Applied Approach

MyPyramid Edition

Janice Thompson
Melinda Manore

Kim Anthony Aaronson

TRUMAN COLLEGE

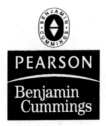

PEARSON

Benjamin
Cummings

San Francisco   Boston   New York
Cape Town   Hong Kong   London   Madrid   Mexico City
Montreal   Munich   Paris   Singapore   Sydney   Tokyo   Toronto

Development Manager: Claire Alexander
Senior Acquisitions Editor: Deirdre Espinoza
Project Editor: Marie Beaugureau
Supplements Production Supervisor: Mary O'Connell
Director of Media Development and Publishing Technology: Lauren Fogel
Managing Editor: Deborah Cogan
Manufacturing Buyer: Stacy Wong
Senior Marketing Manager: Sandra Lindelof
Design and Composition: Elm Street

ISBN 0-8053-8175-9

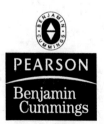

Contents

A User's Guide

Welcome to the study guide to accompany *Nutrition: An Applied Approach, MyPyramid Edition*. By working through this study guide, you will reinforce the concepts covered in your nutrition class.

Here's how the study guide works: The objectives from each chapter of your textbook have been changed into **Investigations** that will guide your learning. As you approach each investigation, you will move through a series of learning exercises that will help you better understand the material. By completing these exercises, the solution to each investigation will unfold. Here are the different types of exercises you will encounter:

Terminology: It is very important to understand the terms used in your textbook to describe concepts in nutrition. In this section, you will define key words from each chapter.

Text Outline Summary: Your textbook has a highly structured organization. This section will help you to see how the material "fits" into the text's organization.

Study Questions: These questions cover all the major topics in a chapter and will bring you closer to the solution to each investigation.

Completion Exercises: These exercises test your understanding of the relationship among different elements in nutrition. Here, you will need to fill in the blanks in a table or on a figure.

Critical Thinking Questions: Once you've covered all the basics, you will be asked to apply your new found knowledge to issues and ideas that your textbook doesn't cover in detail.

Chapter 1

The Role of Nutrition in Our Health

INVESTIGATION 1   What is *nutrition*?

Terminology

Define this term from the text.

Food: _____

TEXT OUTLINE SUMMARY

1.1   What is nutrition?

Study Questions

Answer these questions to develop the solution to the investigation.

Which science studies food? _____

Which science studies how food nourishes our bodies? _____

Which science studies how food influences our health? _____

Completion Exercise

Complete the table below to determine which nutrient stops each disease.

Disease	Discovered when?	Deficient in what nutrient?	Nutrient found in what food?
Scurvy			
Pellagra			

Critical Thinking

Where is it possible to have nutrient deficiency diseases today?

_____

_____

_____

What are some possible causes?

_____

_____

_____

INVESTIGATION 2   Why is *nutrition* important to health?

Terminology

Define each of these terms from the text.

Disease: _____

Health: _____

Wellness: _____

TEXT OUTLINE SUMMARY

1.2   Why is nutrition important?

   1.2.1   Nutrition is one of several factors contributing to wellness.

   1.2.2   A healthful diet can prevent some diseases and reduce your risk for others.

Study Questions

Answer these questions to develop the solution to the investigation.

What was the focus of early research in nutrition? _____

What was the goal of early nutritional science? _____

Adequate nutrient intake in a healthy diet can reduce your risk for what types of diseases?

_____

Completion Exercise

Complete this table using Figure 1.1 in the text.

Wellness Factors

Wellness Factors	Description

Critical Thinking

In the United States, we are facing alarming increases in the number of citizens with obesity, heart disease, type 2 diabetes, stroke, high blood pressure, and cancer. What are the two main factors that individuals can control that could reverse this trend?

_____

_____

_____

INVESTIGATION 3　What are some nutrition-related goals from *Healthy People 2010*?

TEXT OUTLINE SUMMARY

1.2.3　*Healthy People 2010* includes nutrition-related goals for the United States.

Study Questions

Answer these questions to develop the solution to the investigation.

Healthy People 2010 is a _____ promotion and _____ prevention plan for United States citizens.

Completion Exercise

Complete the table below.

Nutrition and Fitness Goals and Objectives from *Healthy People 2010*

Focus Area	Goal	What steps can you take to move toward this goal?
Nutrition and Obesity	Promote health and reduce chronic disease associated with diet and weight.	
Physical Activity and Fitness	Improve health, fitness, and quality of life through daily physical activity.	

Critical Thinking

If the increasing incidence of chronic, debilitating diseases in the United States is not reversed, what are some of the results that might occur to you personally?

_____

_____

_____

INVESTIGATION 4   What are the six classes of nutrients essential for health?

Terminology

Define each of these terms from the text.

Nutrients: _____

Organic: _____

TEXT OUTLINE SUMMARY

1.3   What are nutrients?

Study Questions

Answer these questions to develop the solution to the investigation.

What are organic nutrients? _____

What are inorganic nutrients? _____

Critical Thinking

Would you guess that you need more organic nutrients or more inorganic nutrients in a healthy diet? Explain.

_____

_____

_____

INVESTIGATION 5   What are the three energy nutrients?

Terminology

Define each of these terms from the text.

Kilocalorie: _____

Calorie: _____

Energy: _____

Macronutrients: _____

TEXT OUTLINE SUMMARY

1.3.1   Carbohydrates, fats, and proteins are nutrients that provide energy.

    1.3.1.1   Carbohydrates are a primary fuel source.

    1.3.1.2   Fats provide energy and other essential nutrients.

    1.3.1.3   Proteins support tissue growth, repair, and maintenance.

Study Questions

Answer these questions to develop the solution to the investigation.

Why is alcohol *not* considered an essential nutrient for good health? _____

_____

Why are carbohydrates called carbohydrates? _____

Which nutrient is our *primary* source of energy? _____

What are lipids? _____

Which nutrient group is our *secondary* source of energy? _____

Which nutrient group can be used for energy under extreme conditions, but is more commonly used for growth and repair of body tissues? _____

Completion Exercise

Complete this chart for fats and proteins in this example dietary intake for one day.

Calculating Energy Contribution (Kilocalories) of Carbohydrates, Fats, and Proteins

Nutrient	(kcal/gm)	Amount Consumed in Grams for One Day	Total kcal from This Nutrient Source	Percentage of Total Energy Consumed from This Particular Nutrient Source
Carbohydrates	4	300	1,200	48%
Fats	9	90		
Proteins	4	123		
Totals		513	2,500	100%

Critical Thinking

If a person did not eat for several days, how would he/she get the energy needed to stay alive?

_____

_____

_____

INVESTIGATION 6   What is the difference between vitamins and minerals?

Terminology

Define each of these terms.

Micronutrients: _____

Fat-soluble: _____

Water-soluble: _____

TEXT OUTLINE SUMMARY

1.3.2   Vitamins assist in the regulation of biological processes.

    1.3.2.1   Fat-soluble vitamins are stored in the body.

    1.3.2.2   Water-soluble vitamins should be consumed daily or weekly.

1.3.3   Minerals assist in the regulation of many body functions.

    1.3.3.1   Major minerals are required in amounts greater than 100 milligrams per day.

    1.3.3.2   Trace minerals are required in amounts less than 100 milligrams per day.

1.3.4   Water supports all body functions.

Study Questions

Answer these questions to develop the solution to the investigation.

What are vitamins? _____

What are some of the main functions of vitamins in the body? _____

_____

List the fat-soluble vitamins. _____

List the water-soluble vitamins. _____

Which of these two groups of vitamins can be stored in the body? _____

What are minerals? _____

What is the *main* difference between vitamins and minerals? _____

_____

What is the difference between major minerals and trace minerals? _____

_____

Completion Exercise

Complete this table comparing vitamins and minerals.

Micronutrient	Type	Contain Carbon	Names	Distinguishing Features	Found in These Foods
Vitamins	Fat-soluble	Yes	A, D, E, K		
	Water-soluble	Yes	C, B's		
Minerals	Major	No	calcium, phosphorus, magnesium, sodium, potassium, chloride, sulfur		
	Trace	No	iron, zinc, copper, manganese, selenium, iodine, fluoride, chromium, molybdenum		

Critical Thinking

Which type of vitamins can you take too much of? Why could this happen?

_____

_____

_____

How might it be possible to have an inadequate intake of minerals?

_____

_____

_____

INVESTIGATION 7   What are the Dietary Reference Intakes for nutrients?

Terminology

Define this term from the text.

DRI: _____

TEXT OUTLINE SUMMARY

1.4   How can I figure out my nutrient needs?

    1.4.1   Use the Dietary Reference Intakes to check your nutrient intake.

        1.4.1.1   The Estimated Average Requirement guides the Recommended Dietary Allowance.

        1.4.1.2   The Recommended Dietary Allowance meets the needs of nearly all healthy people.

        1.4.1.3   The Adequate Intake is based on estimates of nutrient intakes.

        1.4.1.4   The Tolerable Upper Intake Level is the highest level that poses no health risk.

        1.4.1.5   The Estimated Energy Requirement is the intake predicted to maintain a healthy weight.

        1.4.1.6   The Acceptable Macronutrient Distribution Ranges are associated with reduced risk for chronic diseases.

    1.4.2   Calculating your unique nutrient needs

Study Questions

Answer these questions to develop the solution to the investigation.

DRIs are dietary standards for _____ people; they do not apply to people with _____ or _____ deficiencies.

Completion Exercise

Complete the table below.

Development of Dietary Reference Intakes (DRIs)

Estimated Average Requirement (ERA)		→		
RDA		→		
AI		→	DRIs for most nutrients →	DRIs Dietary Reference Intakes
UL		→		
EER		→	DRIs for energy and micronutrients →	
AMDR		→		

Critical Thinking

Discuss factors that have a direct impact on a person's actual daily nutrient intake requirements.

_____

_____

_____

INVESTIGATION 8   What are several sources that can provide reliable, accurate nutritional information?

TEXT OUTLINE SUMMARY

1.5   Nutritional advice: Whom can you trust?

    1.5.1   Trustworthy experts are educated and credentialed.

    1.5.2   Government sources of information are usually trustworthy.

    1.5.3   The Centers for Disease Control and Prevention (CDC) protects the health and safety of Americans.

    1.5.4   The National Institutes of Health (NIH) is the leading medical research agency in the world.

    1.5.5   Professional organizations provide reliable nutrition information.

Study Questions

Answer these questions to develop the solution to the investigation.

What is the difference between a licensed nutritionist and a registered dietician?

_____

What is a nutritionist? _____

What is the leading federal agency in the United States that protects the health and safety

of people? _____

Name the world's leading medical research center. _____

Completion Exercise

Complete the table below.

Professional Organizations Providing Accurate Nutritional Information

Abbreviation	Organization Name	Name of Published Journal
ADA		
ASCN		
SNE		
ACSM		

Critical Thinking

Discuss the general trustworthiness of each of the following resources that often cover nutritional topics: TV shows, Web sites, newspapers, magazines, newsletters, and journals.

_____

_____

_____

Medical doctors are generally excellent sources of nutritional and dietary advice. Support or refute this statement with evidence.

_____

_____

_____

Chapter 2

Designing a Healthful Diet

INVESTIGATION 1 What are the components of a healthful diet?

Terminology

Define this term from the text.

Diet: _____

TEXT OUTLINE SUMMARY

2.1   What is a healthful diet?

    2.1.1   A healthful diet is adequate.

    2.1.2   A healthful diet is moderate

    2.1.3   A healthful diet is balanced.

    2.1.4   A healthful diet is varied.

Study Questions

Answer these questions to develop the solution to the investigation.

An adequate diet provides enough _____, _____, and

_____ to maintain health.

What is moderation in a healthful diet? _____

_____

What is balance in a healthful diet? _____

_____

_____

What is variety in a healthful diet? _____

_____

_____

Completion Exercise

Complete the table below showing the components of a healthful diet. (The letters AMBV will help you to remember the four components.)

	Component of a Healthful Diet	Explanation
A	Adequate	
M		Not eating too much or too little of certain foods.
B	Balance	
V		Eating many different foods each day.

Critical Thinking

Why could an adequate diet for one person be inadequate for another?

_____

_____

Would a vegetarian diet be balanced? Explain.

_____

_____

INVESTIGATION 2 How can the nutritional value of a food be determined from the food label?

Terminology

Define this term from the text.

FDA: _____

TEXT OUTLINE SUMMARY

2.2   What tools can help me design a healthful diet?

    2.2.1   Reading food labels can be easy and fun.

        2.2.1.1   Five components must be included on food labels.

            2.2.1.1.1   A statement of identity

            2.2.1.1.2   Net contents of package

            2.2.1.1.3   Ingredient list

            2.2.1.1.4   Name and address of the food manufacturer, packer, or distributor

            2.2.1.1.5   Nutrition information

Study Questions

Answer these questions to develop the solution to the investigation.

What part of a food label can be used to compare one food to another one or to learn more about an individual food?

_____

What are serving sizes?

_____

Percent daily value (%DV) is based on a daily calorie consumption of _____ calories.

Foods containing less than 5%DV of a nutrient are considered _____ in that nutrient.

Foods containing more than 20%DV of a nutrient are considered _____ in that nutrient.

Completion Exercise

Label the five components found on food labels.

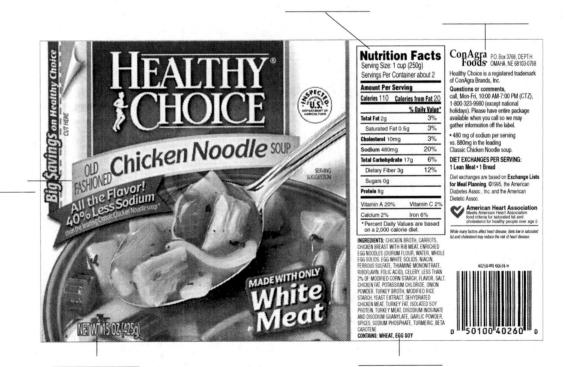

Critical Thinking

How can you determine the percentage of calories that come from fat in a particular food?

_____

_____

To increase your dietary intake of a particular nutrient, how do you know which foods to choose? _____

_____

_____

INVESTIGATION 3 How can the Dietary Guidelines for Americans be used to design a healthful diet?

Terminology

Define this term from the text.

USDHHS: _____

TEXT OUTLINE SUMMARY

2.2.2   Dietary Guidelines for Americans
      2.2.2.1   Adequate nutrients within calorie needs
      2.2.2.2   Weight management
      2.2.2.3   Physical activity
      2.2.2.4   Food groups to encourage
      2.2.2.5   Fats
      2.2.2.6   Carbohydrates
      2.2.2.7   Sodium and potassium
      2.2.2.8   Alcoholic beverages
      2.2.2.9   Food safety

Study Questions

Answer these questions to develop the solution to the investigation.

Which government agencies developed the Dietary Guidelines for Americans 2005?

_____ and _____

What is the purpose of the Dietary Guidelines for Americans 2005? _____

_____

_____

The key to maintaining a healthy weight is to _____ food calories consumed with energy expended.

Moderate physical activity should last at least _____ minutes daily if possible.

List the most common diseases that occur more frequently in overweight individuals.

_____, _____, _____, and _____

Critical Thinking

What role should alcohol play in a healthful diet?

_____

_____

_____

INVESTIGATION 4 What six food groups and serving recommendations are suggested in MyPyramid?

Terminology

Define this term from the text.

USDA: _____

TEXT OUTLINE SUMMARY

    2.2.3   Food Guide Pyramid

        2.2.3.1   What does "serving size" mean in MyPyramid?

        2.2.3.2   Variations of the Food Guide Pyramid

Study Questions

Answer these questions to develop the solution to the investigation. Use www.MyPyramid.gov and your text for your answers.

At least one half of your daily grain intake should be made up of what form of grains?

_____

What should you focus on for your daily fruit and vegetable choices? _____

What is a good source of calcium that should be consumed daily? _____

What foods contain fats that should be consumed daily? _____

What fats should be consumed sparingly? _____

What is a serving of meat? _____

How does a serving of raw vegetables compare to a serving of cooked vegetables?

_____

The number of servings you should consume from each food group is based on

_____

Completion Exercise

Label each one of the rays in MyPyramid with the correct food group.

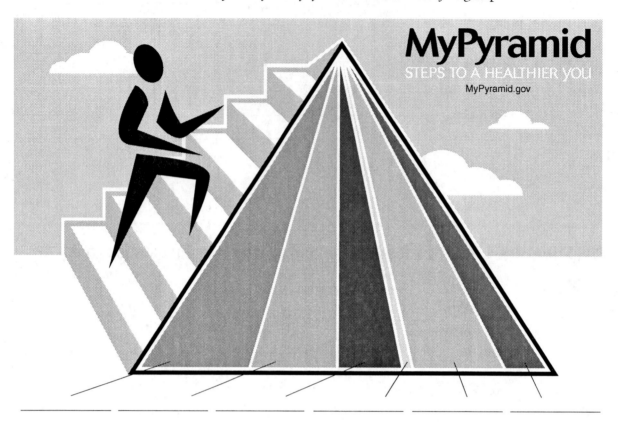

Critical Thinking

How can you consume at least one half of the grains in your diet as whole grains? What changes could you make to accomplish this goal?

_____

_____

_____

INVESTIGATION 5 How can MyPyramid be used to design a healthful diet?

Terminology

Define this term from the text.

Nutrient density: _____

Study Questions

Answer these questions to develop the solution to the investigation.

How can MyPyramid help you to eat an adequate diet? _____

How can MyPyramid help you to eat in moderation? _____

How can MyPyramid help you to eat a balanced diet? _____

In addition to MyPyramid recommendations, what simple strategy can you use to achieve variety in your diet? _____

MyPyramid serving sizes are quite often _____ than food sizes commonly available and consumed.

In response to some of the limitations of the Food Guide Pyramid, Harvard School of Public Health researchers did what? _____

_____

_____

Completion Exercise

Using www.MyPyramid.gov and your text, develop a healthful meal plan for one day in the table below. Build your meals and snacks by indicating the number of servings you will include from each category. Keep your totals for each category in line with your personal MyPyramid recommendations.

Meal	Grains	Vegetables	Fruits	Oils	Milk	Meats and Beans
Breakfast						
Snack						
Lunch						
Snack						
Dinner						
Snack						

Critical Thinking

How could a diet with excessive amounts of food with a low nutrient density adversely affect health?

_____

_____

_____

INVESTIGATION 6 How can the 5-A-Day for The Color Way Program and the DASH plan be used to design a healthful diet?

Terminology

Define each of these terms from the text.

NCI: _____

NIH: _____

DASH: _____

TEXT OUTLINE SUMMARY

    2.2.4   Diet plans

          2.2.4.1   The 5-A-Day The Color Way Program

          2.2.4.2   The DASH diet plan

          2.2.4.3   Other diet plans

Study Questions

Answer these questions to develop the solution to the investigation.

In 1991, why did the National Cancer Institute launch the 5-A-Day The Color Way Program? _____

What is the specific dietary recommendation of the 5-A-Day The Color Way Program?

_____

Why was the DASH diet developed? _____

How is DASH similar to 5-A-Day? _____

What health benefits could occur if all Americans followed the DASH diet?

_____

Critical Thinking

What characteristics of a healthful diet are particularly supported by the 5-A-Day plan?

_____

_____

_____

INVESTIGATION 7 How can the Exchange System be used in a healthful diet?

Terminology

Define this term from the text.

ADA: _____

TEXT OUTLINE SUMMARY

2.2.5 The Exchange System

Study Questions

Answer these questions to develop the solution to the investigation.

How are food exchanges or portions organized in the Exchange System?

_____

List the six major food groups included in the Exchange System.

_____ _____ _____

_____ _____ _____

The Exchange System especially helps to control _____ and

_____ intake.

Completion Exercise

Using Table 2.7 in your text, select and list two possible exchanges for the six specific categories in the table below.

Category	Exchange Choice 1	Exchange Choice 2
Starch/Bread		
Meat (lean)		
Vegetables		
Fruits		
Milk (low fat)		
Fat		

Critical Thinking

What characteristic of a healthful diet is particularly supported by the Exchange System?

_____

_____

_____

INVESTIGATION 8 How can we practice moderation and apply healthful dietary guidelines when eating out?

Text Outline Summary

2.3   Can eating out be part of a healthful diet?

      2.3.1   The hidden costs of eating out

      2.3.2   The healthful way to eat out

Study Questions

Answer these questions to develop the solution to the investigation.

According to the National Restaurant Association, the average American eats out how many times a week? _____

What are several hidden nutritional costs when consuming typical American fast-food meals?

_____

Critical Thinking

Discuss several strategies to maintaining a healthy diet when eating out at a variety of different restaurants.

_____

_____

_____

Chapter 3

The Human Body:
Are We Really What We Eat?

INVESTIGATION 1   What are appetite and hunger and how do they affect our eating?

Terminology

Define each of these terms from the text.

Appetite: _____

Hunger: _____

Hormone: _____

Satiation: _____

TEXT OUTLINE SUMMARY

3.1   Why do we want to eat?

    3.1.1   Food stimulates our senses.

    3.1.2   Psychosocial factors arouse appetite.

    3.1.3   Various factors affect hunger and satiation.

        3.1.3.1   Signals from the brain cause hunger and satiation.

        3.1.3.2   Chemicals called hormones affect hunger and satiation.

        3.1.3.3   The amount and type of food we eat can affect hunger and satiation.

Study Questions

Answer these questions to develop the solution to the investigation.

What is aroused by environmental clues such as the sight or smell of one of your favorite foods? _____

What is related to pleasant sensations related to food? _____

What is the drive that prompts us to find food and to eat? _____

Name some common "triggers" that stimulate appetite. _____

_____

Critical Thinking

What effect would a low blood glucose level have on appetite and hunger?

_____

_____

_____

What effect would a high blood glucose level have on appetite and hunger?

_____

_____

_____

INVESTIGATION 2   Are you really what you eat?

Terminology

Define each of these terms from the text.

Atoms: _____

Molecules: _____

TEXT OUTLINE SUMMARY

3.2   Are we really what we eat?

    3.2.1   Atoms bond to form molecules.

    3.2.2   Food is composed of molecules.

Study Questions

Answer these questions to develop the solution to the investigation.

Atoms connect with other atoms to form _____.

Food and cells are both made up of _____.

Completion Exercise

Complete the table below to determine the makeup of food and humans.

Relative Size	Description	Particle or Unit
Small	The smallest units of matter that cannot be further broken down by any means.	
Slightly Larger in Size	Food we eat is composed of these particles.	
	When food is digested it is then broken down into these particles, which are absorbed into the bloodstream.	
	These particles are then assembled into cellular components to make cells in the human body.	

CRITICAL THINKING

Describe how we "are what we eat" based on molecules.

_____

_____

_____

INVESTIGATION 3   What are the main functions of a cell's plasma membrane?

Terminology

Define each of these terms from the text.

Cell: _____

Cell membrane: _____

TEXT OUTLINE SUMMARY

    3.2.3   Molecules join to form cells.

        3.2.3.1   Cells are encased in a functional membrane.

        3.2.3.2   Cells contain organelles that support life.

    3.2.4   Cells join to form tissues and organs.

Study Questions

Answer these questions to develop the solution to the investigation.

What is the main function of the cell membrane? _____

_____

What is a bilayer? _____

A round phospholipid head connected to a long lipid tail is called a _____.

Completion Exercise

Label this highly magnified portion of a cell (plasma) membrane.

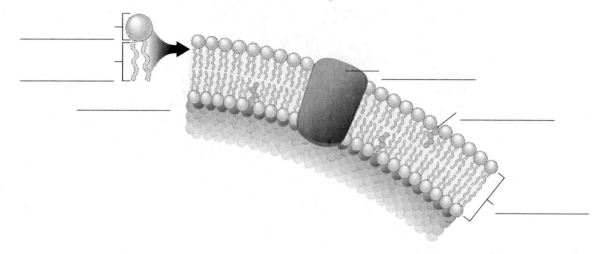

Critical Thinking

The plasma membranes of human cells are selectively permeable. What does this mean and how is it beneficial?

_____

_____

_____

INVESTIGATION 4   Draw a simple diagram of the digestive system and its accessory organs.

Terminology

Define each of these terms from the text.

Tissue: _____

Organ: _____

System: _____

TEXT OUTLINE SUMMARY

3.2.5   Organs make up functional systems.

Study Questions

Answer these questions to develop the solution to the investigation.

The GI tract is made up of the _____ of the _____ system.

List the main organs of the digestive system in order starting with the mouth.

M_____, E_____, S_____,

S_____ I_____, L_____ I_____,

R_____.

List the accessory organs of the digestive system. T_____,

T_____, S_____ G_____,

L_____, G_____b_____, P_____.

Completion Exercise

Complete the labels in the tables below and connect each table box to the correct portion of the diagram.

Accessory Digestive System Organs	Digestive System	Main Organ of the Digestive System
T_____		M_____
T_____		E_____
S_____ G_____		S_____
L_____		S_____ I_____
G_____		L_____ I_____
P_____		R_____

INVESTIGATION 5   How does each digestive organ contribute to the digestion, absorption, and/or elimination of food?

Terminology

Define each of these terms from the text.

Digestion: _____

Absorption: _____

Elimination: _____

3.3   What happens to the food we eat?

     3.3.1   Digestion begins in the mouth.

     3.3.2   The esophagus propels food to the stomach.

     3.3.3   The stomach mixes, digests, and stores food.

     3.3.4   Most digestion and absorption occurs in the small intestine.

         3.3.4.1   The gallbladder and pancreas aid in digestion.

         3.3.4.2   A specialized lining enables the small intestine to absorb food.

         3.3.4.3   Intestinal cells readily absorb vitamins, minerals, and water.

         3.3.4.4   Blood and lymph transport nutrients and fluids.

         3.3.4.5   The liver regulates blood nutrients.

     3.3.5   The large intestine stores food waste until it is excreted.

3.4   How does the body coordinate and regulate digestion?

     3.4.1   The muscles of the gastrointestinal tract mix and move food.

     3.4.2   The enteric nerves coordinate and regulate digestive activities.

Study Questions

Answer these questions to develop the solution to the investigation.

Where does digestion begin? _____

What is the function of the esophagus? _____

What are the three main functions of the stomach? _____,

_____ , and _____ food.

Where does the most food digestion take place? _____

What is the site of most nutrient absorption? _____

What is the site of most water absorption? _____

Completion Exercise

Check the boxes indicating the main function(s) of each main organ of the digestive system.

GI Tract Organs	Digestion (breaking down into absorbable molecules)	Absorption (molecules move into the blood and lymph)	Elimination (nondigestible food is expelled from the body)
Mouth			
Esophagus			
Stomach			
Small Intestine			
Large Intestine			

Critical Thinking

What might occur in the GI tract if peristalsis stopped?

_____

_____

_____

INVESTIGATION 6   What are the main enzymes of digestion and where are they produced?

Terminology

Define this term from the text.

Enzyme: _____

TEXT OUTLINE SUMMARY

See Investigation 5 above.

Study Questions

Answer these questions to develop the solution to the investigation.

Enzymes usually end with what specific letters? _____

Where is the first digestive enzyme in the GI tract found? _____

What is the first digestive enzyme in the GI tract? _____

Name the two main stomach enzymes: _____ and _____ _____

What digestive fluid is released by the gallbladder? _____

Which three enzymes are secreted into the small intestine from the pancreas?

_____ _____, _____ _____, and

_____

Completion Exercise

Complete the table below by indicating the main action of each one of the digestive enzymes or digestive fluids of the GI tract.

Name of Enzyme or Digestive Fluid	Organ Producing the Enzyme or Digestive Fluid	Enzyme or Digestive Fluid Secreted into This Location	Action of Enzyme or Digestive Fluid
Salivary Amylase	Salivary Glands	Mouth	
Hydrochloric Acid	Stomach		
Pepsin			
Gastric Lipase			
Bile	Liver (stored in gallbladder)	Small Intestine	
Pancreatic Lipase	Pancreas		
Pancreatic Amylase			
Pancreatic Proteases			
Bicarbonate			

Critical Thinking

If the stomach did not produce enough HCl (hydrochloric acid), what problem(s) might this cause?

_____

_____

_____

What effect might taking too many antacids have on digestion?

_____

_____

_____

Why do you think scientists have not yet successfully invented an artificial liver?

_____

_____

_____

INVESTIGATION 7   What is GERD? What are ulcers?

Terminology

Define each of these terms from the text.

Reflux: _____

GERD: _____

Peptic ulcer: _____

TEXT OUTLINE SUMMARY

3.5   What disorders are related to digestion, absorption, and elimination?

    3.5.1   Heartburn and gastroesophageal reflux disease (GERD)

    3.5.2   Ulcers

    3.5.3   Food allergies and intolerances

        3.5.3.1   Celiac disease

        3.5.3.2   Food allergies

    3.5.4   Irritable bowel syndrome

Study Questions

Answer these questions to develop the solution to the investigation.

GERD occurs when stomach contents leak "backward" or reflux into which GI tract organ?

_____

Why is this painful? _____

Identify several factors that can aggravate GERD. _____

_____

GI tract ulcers can often be caused by which bacteria? ____

What drugs have a common side effect of causing ulcers? ___

Critical Thinking

If a person always "gulped food down" without chewing it fully, how might this play a role in GERD?

_____

_____

_____

INVESTIGATION 8   What are the main warning signs of dehydration?

Terminology

Define each of these terms from the text, glossary, or other resources.

Diarrhea: _____

Dehydration: _____

Constipation: _____

TEXT OUTLINE SUMMARY

    3.5.5   Diarrhea and constipation

Study Questions

Answer these questions to develop the solution to the investigation.

What is the connection between diarrhea and dehydration? _____

_____

List the most common signs and symptoms of dehydration in adults. _____

_____

List the most common signs and symptoms of dehydration in infants. _____

_____

Critical Thinking

Why is diarrhea so serious in infants?

_____

_____

_____

Chapter 4

Carbohydrates: Bountiful Sources of Energy and Nutrients

INVESTIGATION 1   What is the difference between simple and complex carbohydrates?

Terminology

Define each of these terms from the text.

Photosynthesis: _____

Carbohydrate: _____

Glucose: _____

Monosaccharide: _____

Disaccharide: _____

Polysaccharide: _____

TEXT OUTLINE SUMMARY

4.1   What are carbohydrates?

4.2   What is the difference between simple and complex carbohydrates?

    4.2.1   Glucose, fructose, and galactose are monosaccharides.

    4.2.2   All complex carbohydrates are polysaccharides.

        4.2.2.1   Starch is a polysaccharide stored in plants.

        4.2.2.2   Glycogen is a polysaccharide stored by animals.

        4.2.2.3   Fiber is a polysaccharide that gives plants their structure.

Study Questions

Answer these questions to develop the solution to the investigation.

The simple carbohydrates include the _____ and the _____.

Both of these are also commonly called _____.

What is the most abundant sugar molecule found in our diets and in our bodies and is also the preferred energy source for our brain and body? _____

In nature, glucose is usually found attached to another _____.

What is the sweetest natural sugar that is most commonly found in fruit? _____

By photosynthesis, plants store _____ from the sun in _____ molecules.

Complexes made of long chains of glucose are called _____. The complex carbohydrate produced by plants that is generally digestible in humans is called _____. The complex carbohydrate that stores sugar in humans is called _____. Nondigestible carbohydrates from plants are called _____.

Completion Exercise

Complete the following table showing the composition of simple sugars.

Composition of Simple Sugars		
Monosaccharide	+ Monosaccharide	= Disaccharide
Fructose		Sucrose
Galactose		
Glucose	Glucose	

Critical Thinking

Could you obtain adequate dietary carbohydrates by consuming only sugary drinks like soft drinks and juice cocktails?

_____

_____

_____

INVESTIGATION 2   How are carbohydrates digested and absorbed in our bodies?

Terminology

Define each of these terms from the text.

Dietary fiber: _____

Functional fiber: _____

Total fiber: _____

4.3   How do our bodies break down carbohydrates?

   4.3.1   Digestion breaks down most carbohydrates into monosaccharides.

   4.3.2   The liver converts all disaccharides into glucose.

   4.3.3   Fiber is excreted from the large intestine.

   4.3.4   Insulin and glucagon regulate the level of glucose in our blood.

   4.3.5   The glycemic index shows how foods affect our blood glucose levels.

Study Questions

Answer these questions to develop the solution to the investigation.

Which enzyme breaks down complex carbohydrates (starch) in the mouth? _____

In the mouth, starch is broken down into what molecules? _____

Where does most carbohydrate digestion occur? _____

What enzyme in the small intestine breaks down any remaining starch into disaccharides?

_____

The disaccharides maltose, sucrose, and lactose are digested to monosaccharides by which

three enzymes? _____, _____ and _____

After the monosaccharides are absorbed into the bloodstream, they are all changed to

_____ in the liver. The liver then releases glucose into the bloodstream or

stores the glucose in a complex carbohydrate called _____.

What complex carbohydrate passes out of the body through the GI tract without being

digested? _____

Which two pancreatic hormones regulate the level of glucose in the blood?

_____ and _____

Completion Exercise

Complete the table below.

Starch Digestion

Body Region	Enzyme	Nutrient Acted On	Breakdown Product
Mouth		Starch →	Disaccharides
Small Intestine			Disaccharides
		Sucrose	Monosaccharides (can be absorbed into the blood)
	Lactase		
		Maltose	

Critical Thinking

Why can't humans digest all carbohydrates?

_____

_____

_____

If an individual had severe inflammation of the pancreas, how might this affect carbohydrate digestion?

_____

_____

_____

INVESTIGATION 3   What are the main functions of carbohydrates in our bodies?

TEXT OUTLINE SUMMARY

4.4   Why do we need carbohydrates?

    4.4.1   Carbohydrates provide energy.

        4.4.1.1   Carbohydrates fuel daily activity.

        4.4.1.2   Carbohydrates fuel exercise.

        4.4.1.3   Low carbohydrate intake can lead to ketoacidosis.

        4.4.1.4   Carbohydrates spare protein.

    4.4.2   Complex carbohydrates have health benefits.

    4.4.3   Fiber helps us to stay healthy.

Study Questions

Answer these questions to develop the solution to the investigation.

Carbohydrates provide the main source of _____ for the body.

When carbohydrate intake is inadequate, the body may go into a condition called

_____ that uses fat to provide necessary energy.

Gluconeogenesis makes glucose out of _____ if needed.

Critical Thinking

A long-term diet that contains inadequate fiber may increase the likelihood of which health problems?

_____

_____

_____

INVESTIGATION 4   What are the appropriate intakes for carbohydrates, fiber, and added sugars?

Terminology

Define each of these terms from the text.

RDA: _____

AMDR: _____

TEXT OUTLINE SUMMARY

4.5   How much carbohydrate should we consume?

Study Questions

Answer these questions to develop the solution to the investigation.

How many grams of carbohydrates should be consumed daily just for brain function

alone? _____

What percentage of daily total energy intake should come from carbohydrates? _____

Critical Thinking

What might be the main result of consuming a diet that consistently contains too many carbohydrates?

_____

_____

_____

INVESTIGATION 5   What are some potential health risks with a high intake of simple sugars?

Terminology

Define each of these terms from the text.

Added sugars: _____

Blood lipids: _____

TEXT OUTLINE SUMMARY

4.5.1   Most Americans eat too much simple carbohydrate.

    4.5.1.1   Simple carbohydrates are blamed for many health problems.

    4.5.1.2   Sugar causes tooth decay.

    4.5.1.3   There is no link between sugar and hyperactivity in children.

    4.5.1.4   High sugar intake can lead to unhealthful levels of blood lipids.

    4.5.1.5   High sugar intake does not cause diabetes but may contribute to obesity.

Study Questions

Answer these questions to develop the solution to the investigation.

How does sugar contribute to tooth decay? _____

_____

How does sugar consumption relate to hyperactivity in children? _____

_____

What is the relationship between high sugar consumption and unhealthy blood lipid levels?

_____

How is obesity related to sugar consumption? _____

_____

Critical Thinking

What recommendation would you make to an individual with heart disease regarding his
or her sugar intake?

_____

_____

_____

Why would you make this recommendation?

_____

_____

_____

_____

INVESTIGATION 6   What foods are good sources of carbohydrates?

TEXT OUTLINE SUMMARY

    4.5.2   Most Americans eat too little complex carbohydrate.

        4.5.2.1   We need at least 25 grams of fiber daily.

Study Questions

Answer these questions to develop the solution to the investigation.

What is fiber? _____

What are several good sources of fiber? _____

Fiber is generally found abundantly in what kind of carbohydrates? _____

Completion Exercise

Using Table 4.4 in the textbook, complete the following chart.

List the top four food choices that contain the most fiber in each group. Fill in the grams of fiber per serving for each one of the food choices.

Group	Food	Grams of Fiber/Serving
Vegetables		
Fruits and Juices		
Legumes		
Breads and Cereals		

Critical Thinking

What specific dietary habits cause most Americans to consume too little fiber?

_____

_____

_____

How can you increase the number of complex carbohydrates in your diet?

_____

_____

_____

INVESTIGATION 7 What are the most common alternative sweeteners?

Terminology

Define each of these terms from the text.

Nutritive sweetener: _____

Non-nutritive sweetener: _____

ADI: _____

TEXT OUTLINE SUMMARY

4.6   What is the story on alternative sweeteners?

    4.6.1   Alternative sweeteners are non-nutritive.

    4.6.2   Limited use of alternative sweeteners is not harmful.

        4.6.2.1   Saccharin

            4.6.2.1.1   Acesulfame-K

            4.6.2.1.2   Aspartame

            4.6.2.1.3   Sucralose

            4.6.2.1.4   Other alternative sweeteners

Completion Exercise

Complete the following chart comparing non-nutritive sweeteners using Table 4.6 and your text readings.

Non-Nutritive Sweetener	ADI (mg/kg/day)	How many times sweeter than table sugar (sucrose)?
Saccharin		
Acesulfame-K		
Aspartame (NutraSweet, Equal)		
Sucralose		

Critical Thinking

What possible problems do you see from consuming only non-nutritive sweeteners?

_____

_____

_____

INVESTIGATION 8   What are the types of diabetes and how is diabetes different from hypoglycemia?

Terminology

Define each of these terms from the text, glossary, or other resources.

Type 1 diabetes: _____

Type 2 diabetes: _____

Hyperglycemia: _____

Hypoglycemia: _____

TEXT OUTLINE SUMMARY

4.7   What disorders are related to carbohydrate metabolism?

    4.7.1   Diabetes; impaired glucose regulation

        4.7.1.1   In type 1 diabetes the body does not produce enough insulin.

        4.7.1.2   In type 2 diabetes the cells become less responsive to insulin.

        4.7.1.3   Lifestyle choices can help control or prevent diabetes.

    4.7.2   Hypoglycemia: low blood glucose

    4.7.3.   Lactose intolerance: inability to digest lactose

Study Questions

Answer these questions to develop the solution to the investigation.

What is another name for type 1 diabetes? _____

What is the main problem for the patient with type 1 diabetes? _____

_____

What is another name for type 2 diabetes? _____

What is the main problem for the patient with type 2 diabetes? _____

_____

What is the main cause of hypoglycemia? _____

_____

An individual who is lactose intolerant is not producing enough _____

Critical Thinking

What dietary and lifestyle recommendations would you suggest to an individual with type 2 diabetes?

_____

_____

_____

Chapter 5

Fat: An Essential Energy-Supplying Nutrient

INVESTIGATION 1   What are the three most common types of lipids found in foods?

Terminology

Define each of these terms from the text.

Lipid: _____

Triglyceride: _____

Fatty acid: _____

Glycerol: _____

Phospholipid: _____

Sterol: _____

TEXT OUTLINE SUMMARY

5.1   What are fats?

    5.1.1   Lipids come in different forms.

    5.1.2   Three types of lipids are present in foods.

        5.1.2.1   Triglycerides are the most common food-based lipid.

        5.1.2.2   Phospholipids combine lipids with phosphates.

        5.1.2.3   Sterols have a ring structure.

Study Questions

Answer these questions to develop the solution to the investigation.

Fats and oils belong to a group of substances called _____.

Most lipids are _____ in water.

What are the three types of lipids found in food? _____, _____,

and _____

Which of the three types of lipids is most often found in food? _____

A triglyceride is made of three _____ attached to a three-carbon glycerol

_____ .

A phospholipid is made of two _____ and a phosphate compound attached

to a glycerol _____ .

Which one of the lipids has a carbon-ring structure? _____

Critical Thinking

Discuss the similarities and differences between triglycerides and phospholipids.

_____

_____

_____

INVESTIGATION 2   How does saturation affect the shape or form of saturated fats?

Terminology

Define each of these terms from the text.

SFA: _____

MUFA: _____

PUFA: _____

TEXT OUTLINE SUMMARY

     5.1.2.4   Triglycerides are classified by their length, saturation, and shape.

         5.1.2.4.1   Chain length

         5.1.2.4.2   Level of saturation

Study Questions

Answer these questions to develop the solution to the investigation.

Fatty acids consist of a chain of _____ atoms with many attached

_____ atoms. A chain of carbon atoms is "saturated" with _____

atoms if there are two attached to each carbon atom in the chain. In a MUFA chain, one

set of two adjacent carbon atoms is attached together with a _____ bond.

Each one of these two adjacent carbons has only _____ hydrogen atom at-

tached, and is therefore "unsaturated." These two hydrogen atoms tend to attach on the

same side of the carbon chain, resulting in a "bend" in the chain. Bent molecules cannot

stack _____ together, so MUFAs tend to be liquid at room temperature.

PUFAs have two or more sets of _____, double-bonded carbon atoms. PUFAs are also _____ at room temperature. Saturated fatty acid chains have two _____ atoms attached to each carbon and result in a carbon chain with _____ bends. SFA molecules can lie closely together, resulting in saturated fats being _____ at room temperature.

Completion Exercise

Complete the following table comparing fatty acids.

Type of FA	Number of C=C bonds	Molecule Shape	Room Temperature State
SFA		Straight	
MUFA			Liquid
PUFA	Two or more		

Critical Thinking

Coconut oil is solid below 76 degrees F and is liquid above 76 degrees F. What type of fatty acids do you predict make up this unique oil?

_____

_____

_____

INVESTIGATION 3   What is the difference between *cis* and *trans* fats?

Terminology

Define each of these terms from the text.

Cis: _____

Trans: _____

TEXT OUTLINE SUMMARY

        5.1.2.4.3   Shape

                5.1.2.4.3.1 *Cis*

                5.1.2.4.3.2 *Trans*

Study Questions

Answer these questions to develop the solution to the investigation.

MUFAs contain one C=C bond with each C having a _____ attached on the same side in the _____ configuration. This results in MUFAs having a bent shape, which contributes to their being in a _____ state at room temperature. This shape is commonly found in natural foods. When MUFAs or PUFAs are hydrogenated during processing, some of the hydrogen atoms attach on opposite sides of the C=C unsaturated bond. This is called the _____ position and results in some MUFA or PUFA molecules having a straight shape. As a result, these *trans* fats are _____ at room temperature. This shape is rarely found in natural foods.

Critical Thinking

Trans fats are chemically "unsaturated" yet they are in a solid state like "saturated" fats. How might this deception affect the body's fat digestion and utilization?

_____

_____

_____

INVESTIGATION 4   How is fat digested?

Terminology

Define each of these terms from the text.

Bile: _____

Monoglyceride: _____

Lipoprotein: _____

Chylomicron: _____

LPL: _____

TEXT OUTLINE SUMMARY

5.2   How does our body break down fats?

    5.2.1   The gallbladder, liver, and pancreas assist in fat digestion.

    5.2.2   Absorption of fat occurs primarily in the small intestine.

    5.2.3   Fat is stored in adipose tissue for later use.

Study Questions

Answer these questions to develop the solution to the investigation.

Where does most fat digestion and absorption occur? _____

Bile is produced in the _____ and stored in the _____ .

When is bile released into the small intestine? _____

How does bile aid fat digestion? _____

Because fat is not water soluble, it must be packaged by the small intestine into a special

lipoprotein molecule called a _____, which can then be absorbed into

the lymph and into the blood.

What makes lipoproteins water soluble? _____

How does the fat in a chylomicron in the bloodstream get into a fat cell (in adipose tissue)

in the body? _____

Completion Exercise

Using Figure 5.6 in the text, indicate what occurs to dietary fats in each of the four locations of the digestive system.

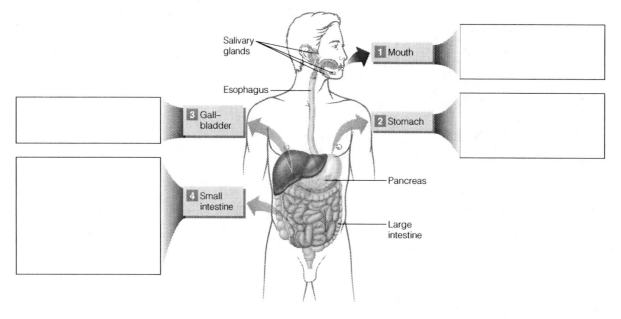

Critical Thinking

If a person has had his or her gallbladder removed (cholecystectomy), what dietary advice would you give that person and why?

_____

_____

_____

INVESTIGATION 5 What are the three main functions of fat in our body?

Terminology

Define each of these terms from the text.

EFA: _____

Omega-6 fatty acid: _____

Omega-3 fatty acid: _____

TEXT OUTLINE SUMMARY

5.3   Why do we need fats?

    5.3.1   Fats provide energy.

        5.3.1.1   Fats are a major fuel source when we are at rest.

        5.3.1.2   Fats fuel physical activity.

    5.3.2   Fats store energy for later use.

    5.3.3   Fats provide essential fatty acids.

        5.3.3.1   Linoleic acid (omega-6 fatty acid)

        5.3.3.2   Alpha-linolenic acid (omega-3 fatty acid)

            5.3.3.2.1   Eicosapentaenoic acid (EPA)

            5.3.3.2.2   Docosahexaenoic acid (DHA)

    5.3.4   Fats enable the transport of fat-soluble vitamins.

    5.3.5   Fats help maintain cell function and provide protection to the body.

    5.3.6   Fats contribute to the flavor and texture of food.

        5.3.6.1   Fats help us to feel satiated.

5.4   When are fats harmful?

    5.4.1   Eating too much of certain fats can lead to disease.

    5.4.2   Fats limit the shelf life of foods.

Study Questions

Answer these questions to develop the solution to the investigation.

What makes fats such a good energy source? _____

Exercise causes the release of adrenaline. How does this affect using fat for energy?

_____

What role does exercise play in using fat for energy? _____

People who regularly exercise generally have _____ subcutaneous adipose tissue than do "couch potatoes." Fats that cannot be made in the body and must be consumed in the diet are called _____ fats. Dietary fats also assist in the efficient absorption of _____-soluble vitamins such as vitamins _____,

_____, _____, and _____.

Completion Exercise

Complete the following chart to increase your understanding of essential fatty acids.

Main EFAs	Subgroups	Other Name	Function	Sources
Linoleic	none	omega-6	regulation	
Alpha-linolenic	EPA			vegetable oils, fish, and fish oils
	DHA			

Critical Thinking

Can a person obtain an appropriate amount of EFAs if he or she never eats fish or vegetable oil that has not been used for frying?

_____

_____

_____

INVESTIGATION 6   How much total fat, saturated fat, and essential fatty acids should we eat every day?

Terminology

Define this term from the text.

AMDR: _____

TEXT OUTLINE SUMMARY

5.5   How much fat should we eat?

    5.5.1   Dietary reference intake for total fat

    5.5.2   Dietary reference intakes for essential fatty acids

    5.5.3   Most Americans eat within the recommended amount of fat but eat the wrong types.

Study Questions

Answer these questions to develop the solution to the investigation.

What percent of your total energy intake per day should come from fat? _____

Which fats should be decreased in a healthy diet? _____

Athletes should consume _____ fat than the average person.

Of the total AMDR for daily fat intake, what percentage should come from omega-6 fats and what percentage from omega-3 fats? _____ and _____

Critical Thinking

What are some reasons that Americans consume so much saturated and *trans* fats?

_____

_____

_____

How can you decrease your consumption of saturated and *trans* fats?

_____

_____

_____

INVESTIGATION 7   What are some common food sources of beneficial fats?

Terminology

Define this term from the text.

Invisible fats: _____

TEXT OUTLINE SUMMARY

    5.5.4   Shopper's guide: food sources of fat
        5.5.4.1   Visible versus invisible fats
        5.5.4.2   Food sources of beneficial fats
        5.5.4.3   Fat replacers

Study Questions

Answer these questions to develop the solution to the investigation.

Many processed foods contain _____ sources of fat and these are often

_____ or _____ fats.

Many whole foods such as oils, nuts, and fish are rich sources of _____ oils

that our bodies need.

Completion Exercise

Use Table 5.1 in the text to complete the following chart by choosing the top three sources of dietary fat in each category.

Highest % of Total Calories from Fat	Highest % of Total Calories from EFAs	Highest % of Total Calories from PUFAs	Highest % of Total Calories from MUFAs	Highest % of Total Calories from SFAs

Critical Thinking

How can you increase your consumption of good fats in your diet?

_____

_____

_____

INVESTIGATION 8   How does dietary fat intake affect the development of cardiovascular disease?

Terminology

Define each of these terms from the text.

Cardiovascular disease: _____

VLDL: _____

LDL: _____

HDL: _____

TEXT OUTLINE SUMMARY

5.6   What health problems are related to fat intake or metabolism?

    5.6.1   Fats can protect against or promote cardiovascular disease.

        5.6.1.1   Risk factors for cardiovascular disease

            5.6.1.1.1   Overweight

            5.6.1.1.2   Physical inactivity

            5.6.1.1.3   Smoking

            5.6.1.1.4   High blood pressure

            5.6.1.1.5   Diabetes mellitus

        5.6.1.2   Calculating your risk for cardiovascular disease

        5.6.1.3   The role of dietary fats in cardiovascular disease

        5.6.1.4   Lifestyle changes can prevent or reduce cardiovascular disease.

    5.6.2   Does a high-fat diet cause cancer?

Study Questions

Answer these questions to develop the solution to the investigation.

Blood lipids are another name for _____ in the blood.

Which blood lipid contains the most protein? _____

Which blood lipid contains the most cholesterol? _____

A diet containing a lot of saturated fat, simple sugars, and extra calories will result in elevated levels of which blood lipid? _____

Adequate consumption of omega-3 fatty acids in the diet reduces the level of what blood lipid? _____

What is the "good" blood lipid? _____

Completion Exercise

Use Figure 5.13 in the text to complete the following chart comparing the various blood lipids.

	Protein	Phospholipids	Triglycerides	Cholesterol
Chylomicron				
VLDL				
LDL				
HDL				

Critical Thinking

What kind of dietary and lifestyle changes could you adopt to decrease your likelihood of developing cardiovascular disease?

_____

_____

_____

Specifically, what foods will you decrease or avoid in your diet?

_____

_____

_____

Specifically, what foods will you increase in your diet?

_____

_____

_____

Chapter 6

Proteins: Crucial Components of All Body Tissues

INVESTIGATION 1   How do proteins differ from carbohydrates and fats?

Terminology

Define each of these terms from the text.

Protein: _____

Carbohydrate: _____

Fat: _____

Amino acid: _____

Essential amino acid: _____

DNA: _____

Peptide: _____

Polypeptide: _____

Synthesis: _____

TEXT OUTLINE SUMMARY

6.1   What are proteins?

     6.1.1   How do proteins differ from carbohydrates and lipids?

     6.1.2   The building blocks of proteins are amino acids.

         6.1.2.1   We must obtain essential amino acids from food.

         6.1.2.2   Our bodies can make nonessential amino acids.

6.2   How are proteins made?

     6.2.1   Amino acids bond to form a variety of peptides.

         6.2.1.1   Genes regulate amino acid binding.

         6.2.1.2   Amino acid binding and attraction determine shape.

     6.2.2   Protein shape determines function.

     6.2.3   Protein synthesis can be limited by missing amino acids.

     6.2.4   Protein synthesis can be enhanced by mutual supplementation.

Study Questions

Answer these questions to develop the solution to the investigation.

What three elements are found in proteins, carbohydrates, and fats? _____,

_____, and _____

Proteins also contain a very usable form of what additional element? _____

Proteins are synthesized building blocks called _____.

Nonessential amino acids can be _____ by the body.

Essential amino acids must be _____ in the diet.

The directions to build specific proteins are contained in the _____ found in the cell nucleus.

Completion Exercise

Complete the following diagram showing how proteins are built from amino acids.

1. _____	6. _____
2. _____	7. _____
3. _____	8. _____
4. _____	9. _____
5. _____	10. _____

Critical Thinking

Shape determines function in proteins . If there is a mistake in the sequence coding for hemoglobin, what effect might this have on the shape of the resulting hemoglobin molecule?

_____

_____

_____

What effect would this have on the function of this particular kind of hemoglobin?

_____

_____

_____

INVESTIGATION 2   What nonmeat food combinations together provide complete protein?

Terminology

Define each of these terms from the text.

Incomplete proteins: _____

Complete proteins: _____

Complementary proteins: _____

Mutual supplementation: _____

Study Questions

Answer these questions to develop the solution to the investigation.

A protein that contains all of the essential amino acids is called a(n) _____ protein.

A protein that does not contain all of the essential amino acids is called a(n) _____ protein.

If two protein food sources are missing different essential amino acids, these two foods are _____ to each other.

If two protein food sources that are missing different essential amino acids are consumed together, this process is called _____ supplementation and results in a complete dietary protein.

Completion Exercise

Complete the table below on how to obtain complete dietary protein by mutual supplementation.

Most prominent food in a meal	Complete or incomplete protein?	Missing what essential amino acids?	Complementary food(s) that can be added to the food in the first column to make the dietary protein for the meal complete
Rice (grains)			
Beans (legumes)			
Vegetables			
Beef			

Critical Thinking

In many cultures beans and rice are frequently consumed together. Why is this specific combination of foods excellent nutritionally?

_____

_____

_____

Would a diet composed only of fruits and vegetables be adequate for good nutrition? Explain.

_____

_____

_____

INVESTIGATION 3   How are proteins digested and absorbed by our bodies?

Terminology

Define each of these terms from the text.

Hydrochloric acid: _____

Pepsinogen: _____

Pepsin: _____

Enzymes: _____

Proteases: _____

TEXT OUTLINE SUMMARY

6.3   How do our bodies break down proteins?

    6.3.1   Stomach acids and enzymes break proteins into short polypeptides.

    6.3.2   Enzymes in the small intestine break polypeptides into single amino acids.

    6.3.3   Protein digestibility affects protein quality.

Study Questions

Answer these questions to develop the solution to the investigation.

What happens to proteins in the mouth? _____

_____

What happens to proteins in the stomach? _____

_____

What happens to proteins in the small intestine? _____

_____

What protein molecules are absorbed into cells in the wall of the small intestine?

_____ , _____ , and _____

Enzymes in the cells of the small intestine's walls break down all polypeptides into

_____ , which are then absorbed into the bloodstream and transported

to the _____ and then to whatever cells in the body need them.

Completion Exercise

Complete the following chart on protein digestion. Use Figure 6.6 in the text as a reference.

Digestive System Organ	Liquid Secretion (if any)	What happens to protein?
Mouth		
Stomach		
Small intestine		
Small intestine lining cells		

Critical Thinking

What effect would taking antacids have on protein digestion?

_____

_____

_____

How is digestibility significant when determining the quality of a particular protein?

_____

_____

_____

Rank the following foods in order of digestibility, from most digestible (1) to least digestible (4), and explain why you put them in that particular order: well-done steak, raw peas, cooked peas, raw steak.

1. _____ _____

_____

2. _____ _____

_____

3. _____ _____

_____

4. _____ _____

_____

INVESTIGATION 4   What are four main functions of proteins in our bodies?

Terminology

Define each of these terms from the text.

Enzymes: _____

Hormones: _____

Insulin: _____

Electrolytes: _____

Edema: _____

pH: _____

Acidosis: _____

Alkalosis: _____

Buffers: _____

Antibodies: _____

Deamination: _____

Urea: _____

TEXT OUTLINE SUMMARY

6.4   Why do we need proteins?

    6.4.1   Proteins contribute to cell growth, repair, and maintenance.

    6.4.2   Proteins act as enzymes and hormones.

    6.4.3   Proteins help maintain fluid and electrolyte balance.

    6.4.4   Proteins help maintain acid-base balance.

    6.4.5   Proteins help maintain a strong immune system.

    6.4.6   Proteins serve as an energy source.

Study Questions

Answer these questions to develop the solution to the investigation.

What cells inside our body are replaced most frequently? _____

How often are these cells replaced? _____

What hormone produced by the pancreas helps body cells to take in glucose? _____

How do transport proteins maintain the electrolyte levels inside cells? _____

_____

Proteins in the body act as _____ that minimize acid-base shifts in the

blood and thus help to maintain homeostasis.

Why does a person ill with a bacterial infection need adequate protein intake? _____

_____

When would protein be used as a source of energy for the body? _____

_____

Completion Exercise

Label each one of the components of an enzyme reaction in this diagram. Use Figure 6.7 from the text as a reference.

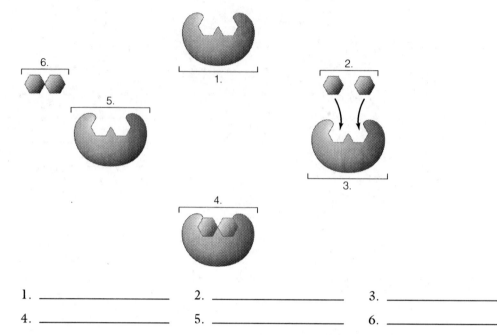

1. _____   2. _____   3. _____

4. _____   5. _____   6. _____

Critical Thinking

Compare and contrast growth and repair.

_____

_____

_____

Who would need more protein, an Olympic athlete or a couch potato? Explain your reasoning.

_____

_____

_____

List several specific instances during adulthood when protein needs would increase.

_____

_____

_____

INVESTIGATION 5   How much protein should you consume every day?

Terminology

Define this term from the text.

RDA: _____

TEXT OUTLINE SUMMARY

6.5   How much protein should we eat?

    6.5.1   Recommended dietary allowance (RDA) for protein

    6.5.2   Most Americans meet or exceed the RDA for protein.

Study Questions

Answer this question to develop the solution to the investigation.

How much of your daily dietary energy (food) intake should come from protein?

_____%

Calculate Your Personal Protein Needs

Take your weight in pounds (_____) and divide by 2.2 to get your weight in

kilograms (_____). Multiply your weight in kilograms by 0.8 and enter that

number here _____ .

This is the number of grams of protein you should consume per day. Adjust the 0.8 as

necessary depending on your activity level.

Critical Thinking

Bodybuilders have a much greater RDA for protein than other athletes. List several reasons why this is true.

_____

_____

_____

Eating extra protein will not make a person's muscles larger. Why not?

_____

_____

_____

Taking the above two questions into consideration, what would you recommend to someone who has just retired from a job that required daily heavy labor with regard to RDA for protein?

_____

_____

_____

INVESTIGATION 6 What potential health risks may be associated with high-protein diets?

Terminology

Define each of these terms from the text.

Cholesterol: _____

Calcium: _____

Acidic: _____

TEXT OUTLINE SUMMARY

6.5.3 Too much dietary protein can be harmful.

    6.5.3.1 High-protein intake is associated with high cholesterol.

    6.5.3.2 High-protein intake may contribute to bone loss.

    6.5.3.3 High-protein intake can increase the risk for kidney disease.

Study Questions

Answer these questions to develop the solution to the investigation.

What is the relationship between high animal protein consumption and blood cholesterol

levels? _____

High-protein diets increase _____ excretion in the urine, which may

contribute to bone loss.

High-protein intake leads to increased protein metabolism, causing higher levels of

_____ production. Adequate fluid intake is needed to flush this excess

_____ through the kidneys.

Critical Thinking

What suggestion about protein intake would you make to an individual with kidney disease?

_____

_____

_____

What suggestion about protein intake would you make to an individual with severe kidney disease who is on dialysis?

_____

_____

_____

INVESTIGATION 7   What foods are good sources of protein?

Terminology

Define this term from the text.

Legume: _____

TEXT OUTLINE SUMMARY

6.5.4   Shopper's guide: good food sources of protein

6.5.5   Can a vegetarian diet provide adequate protein?

    6.5.5.1   Types of vegetarian diets

    6.5.5.2   Why do people become vegetarians?

        6.5.5.2.1   Religious, ethical, and food-safety reasons

        6.5.5.2.2   Ecological benefits

        6.5.5.2.3   Health benefits

    6.5.5.3   What are the challenges of a vegetarian diet?

    6.5.5.4   Using the Vegetarian Food Guide Pyramid to achieve the RDA for protein

Study Questions

Answer these questions to develop the solution to the investigation.

The best dietary sources of protein include _____

and _____ products.

An excellent nonmeat source of protein is found in the group of foods called

_____, which includes beans.

Name several legume sources of protein. _____

_____

Completion Exercise

Using Table 6.5 in the text, complete the following chart indicating your favorite food protein source from each of the main groups (where applicable to your diet).

Group	Your Favorite Food Choice	Serving Size	Grams of Protein/Serving
Beef			
Poultry			
Seafood			
Pork			
Dairy products			
Soy products			
Beans			
Nuts			
Cereals, grains			
Breads			
Vegetables			

Critical Thinking

Which major food group is missing from the table above?

_____

_____

_____

Why is this group absent?

_____

_____

_____

INVESTIGATION 8 What are the main disorders related to inadequate protein intake or genetic abnormalities?

Terminology

Define each of these terms from the text, glossary, or other resources.

Protein-energy malnutrition: _____

Anemia: _____

Edema: _____

TEXT OUTLINE SUMMARY

6.6 What disorders are related to protein intake or metabolism?

    6.6.1 Protein-energy malnutrition can lead to debility and death.

        6.6.1.1 Marasmus results from grossly inadequate energy intake.

        6.6.1.2 Kwashiorkor results from a low-protein diet.

    6.6.2 Disorders related to genetic abnormalities

        6.6.2.1 Sickle cell anemia

        6.6.2.2 Cystic fibrosis

Study Questions

Answer these questions to develop the solution to the investigation.

Inadequate intake of all nutrients can lead to the "skin-and-bones" appearance of the disease called _____.

Infants who are suddenly weaned from breast milk and fed a thin, cereal gruel can quickly develop the swollen-stomach appearance of _____. In this condition fluid and electrolyte imbalances result in extreme distension of the belly, which is called _____.

Both of the above conditions are examples of _____-_____ malnutrition.

Genetic defects occur when an individual's _____, or genetic blueprint, is defective.

The enzyme necessary to break down phenylalanine is absent in an individual with

_____.

In a person with the genetic abnormality that results in sickle cell anemia, the hemoglobin molecules in the red blood cells are _____ shaped.

An abnormal protein that prevents the normal movement of chloride into and out of certain cells is found in the genetic condition called _____ _____.

Critical Thinking

If you were to provide relief foodstuffs to reverse marasmus, what foods would you focus on providing?

_____

_____

_____

If you were to provide relief foodstuffs to reverse kwashiorkor, what foods would you focus on providing?

_____

_____

_____

Chapter 7

Nutrients Involved in Fluid and Electrolyte Balance

INVESTIGATION 1   What are the four most common nutrients that function as electrolytes in our bodies?

Terminology

Define each of these terms from the text.

Fluid: _____

Intracellular: _____

Extracellular: _____

Electrolyte: _____

TEXT OUTLINE SUMMARY

7.1.   What are fluids and electrolytes and what are their functions?

    7.1.1   Body fluid is the liquid portion of our cells and tissues.

        7.1.1.1   Intracellular fluid

        7.1.1.2   Extracellular fluid

            7.1.1.2.1   Tissue (interstitial) fluid

            7.1.1.2.2   Plasma

    7.1.2   Body fluid is composed of water and dissolved substances called electrolytes.

Study Questions

Answer these questions to develop the solution to the investigation.

Approximately how much of your body weight is fluid? _____

How much of this body fluid is found within cells (intracellular)? _____

What are the two main types of extracellular fluid? _____

and _____ (also known as interstitial fluid)

Body fluid is composed of water and dissolved substances called _____.

What are the four main minerals that act as electrolytes in our body? _____,

_____, _____, and _____

How do electrolytes usually enter the body? _____

Completion Exercise

Complete the following table comparing the four main electrolytes.

Mineral Name	Symbol	Charge	Forms This Ion in the Body	Most Common Location	
				Intracellular	Extracellular
Sodium					X
Potassium				X	
Chloride					X
Phosphorus			$H_2PO_4^{-2}$	X	

Critical Thinking

What would you predict would occur to the electrolyte levels in the body fluids as a person became more and more dehydrated?

_____

_____

_____

INVESTIGATION 2   What are the four main functions of water in our bodies?

Terminology

Define this term from the text.

Solvent: _____

TEXT OUTLINE SUMMARY

7.1.3   Fluids serve many critical functions.

    7.1.3.1   Fluids dissolve and transport substances.

    7.1.3.2   Fluids account for blood volume.

    7.1.3.3   Fluids help maintain body temperature.

    7.1.3.4   Fluids protect and lubricate our tissues.

Study Questions

Answer these questions to develop the solution to the investigation.

List the common water-soluble substances that are carried throughout the body in the

blood. _____, _____, _____, and

_____

Adequate _____ intake is necessary to maintain normal blood volume.

Blood volume that is too low can cause _____ blood pressure, which is also called _____.

Water temperature tends to remain stable because water has a high _____ _____, meaning it takes a lot of energy to raise the water temperature. This makes body fluids very helpful in maintaining normal _____ temperature.

Cerebrospinal fluid (CSF) around the brain and spinal cord provides _____.

Synovial fluid found in movable, cartilaginous joints provides _____.

Critical Thinking

Thinking of body fluids, particularly blood volume, what dietary suggestion might be helpful for a person with high blood pressure?

_____

_____

_____

If a body cell is placed in pure water, what do you think will happen and why?

_____

_____

_____

Why is it better to use normal saline to wash your eyes rather than plain water?

_____

_____

_____

INVESTIGATION 3   How do electrolytes help in regulating a healthful fluid balance?

Terminology

Define this term from the text.

Permeable: _____

TEXT OUTLINE SUMMARY

7.1.4   Electrolytes support many body functions.

7.1.4.1   Electrolytes help regulate fluid balance.

7.1.4.2   Electrolytes enable our nerves to respond to stimuli.

7.1.4.3   Electrolytes signal our muscles to contract.

Study Questions

Answer these questions to develop the solution to the investigation.

Cell membranes in our body are _____ to water and are not freely

_____ to electrolytes.

In our body, water always flows where _____ are present.

Body cells can efficiently regulate the amount of water in cells by actively pumping

_____ across cell membranes.

Using Figure 7.4 in the text, answer the following two questions:

Why did the water move to the salt side of the glass? _____

_____

Why didn't the salt move to the other side of the glass? _____

_____

Critical Thinking

What effect would severe diarrhea have on intracellular and extracellular water balance in the body?

_____

_____

_____

INVESTIGATION 4 What physical changes occur in our body to cause us to become thirsty?

Terminology

Define each of these terms from the text.

Thirst: _____

Hypothalamus: _____

Thirst mechanism: _____

TEXT OUTLINE SUMMARY

7.2   How do our bodies maintain fluid balance?

  7.2.1   Our thirst mechanism prompts us to drink fluids.

Study Questions

Answer these questions to develop the solution to the investigation.

The thirst mechanism located in the _____ in the brain responds to particular

body changes by making us thirsty and causing us to drink to reverse those changes.

Eating a lot of salty foods makes us thirsty because of a high level of _____ in our blood after eating these foods.

If blood volume and blood pressure _____, thirst results.

Name five ways that blood volume could decrease. _____, _____, _____, _____, and _____

Tissue dryness in the _____ leads to increased production of saliva and thirst.

Critical Thinking

At the same time our thirst mechanism is stimulated, what beneficial change occurs in the kidney to help conserve water?

_____

_____

_____

INVESTIGATION 5   How do fluids get into and out of our bodies?

Terminology

Define each of these terms from the text.

Metabolic water: _____

Insensible: _____

Insensible water loss: _____

Diuretic: _____

TEXT OUTLINE SUMMARY

7.2.2   We gain fluids by consuming beverages and foods and through metabolism.

7.2.3   We lose fluids through urine, sweat, exhalation, and feces.

Study Questions

Answer these questions to develop the solution to the investigation.

What is the most common way we get water into our bodies? _____

Metabolism (digestion) of _____ also puts water into our bodies.

What is the most common way that fluids leave the body? _____

Insensible water loss occurs through _____ and _____.

Some water is normally excreted through our intestines in our _____.

Completion Exercise

Complete the following diagram showing water balance in the body through fluid intake and output.

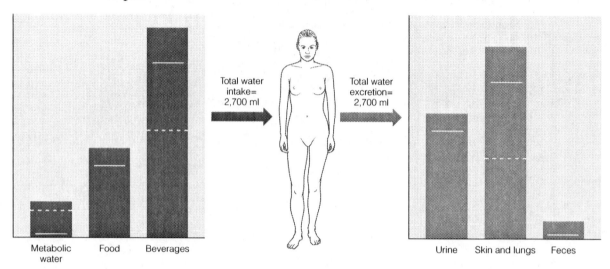

Total water intake= 2,700 ml

Total water excretion= 2,700 ml

Metabolic water   Food   Beverages

Urine   Skin and lungs   Feces

Critical Thinking

Why might a person be told by a physician to take diuretics?

_____

_____

_____

How could you use the information in Table 7.1 from the text to increase your daily water intake?

_____

_____

_____

How does consuming alcohol affect the body's water balance?

_____

_____

_____

INVESTIGATION 6 What is hyponatremia and how is it caused?

Terminology

Define each of these terms from the text.

Hypernatremia: _____

Hyponatremia: _____

Hyperkalemia: _____

Hypokalemia: _____

TEXT OUTLINE SUMMARY

7.3   A profile of nutrients involved in hydration and neuromuscular function

     7.3.1   Water

         7.3.1.1   How much water should we drink?

             7.3.1.1.1   Recommended intake

         7.3.1.2   Sources of drinking water

         7.3.1.3   What happens if we drink too much water?

         7.3.1.4   What happens if we don't drink enough water?

     7.3.2   Sodium

         7.3.2.1   Functions of sodium

         7.3.2.2   How much sodium should we consume?

             7.3.2.2.1   Recommended dietary intake for sodium

                 7.3.2.2.1.1   Good food sources of sodium

         7.3.2.3   What happens if we consume too much sodium?

         7.3.2.4   What happens if we don't consume enough sodium?

     7.3.3   Potassium

         7.3.3.1   Functions of potassium

         7.3.3.2   How much potassium should we consume?

             7.3.3.2.1   Recommended dietary intake for potassium

                 7.3.3.2.1.1   Good food sources of potassium

         7.3.3.3   What happens if we consume too much potassium?

         7.3.3.4   What happens if we don't consume enough potassium?

     7.3.4   Chloride

         7.3.4.1   Functions of chloride

         7.3.4.2   How much chloride should we consume?

         7.3.4.3   What happens if we consume too much chloride?

         7.3.4.4   What happens if we don't consume enough chloride?

     7.3.5   Phosphorus

         7.3.5.1   Functions of phosphorus

         7.3.5.2   How much phosphorus should we consume?

         7.3.5.3   What happens if we consume too much phosphorus?

         7.3.5.4   What happens if we don't consume enough phosphorus?

Study Questions

Answer these questions to develop the solution to the investigation.

Consuming too much NaCl (table salt) can result in an abnormally elevated Na^+ level in the blood, which is called _____.

Inadequate Na^+ intake or replacement results in a low Na^+ level in the blood, which is called _____.

What are the common deficiency symptoms of hyponatremia? _____

_____

_____

How can hyponatremia be treated and/or prevented? _____

_____

Critical Thinking

Why do athletes sometimes take "salt tablets"?

_____

_____

_____

What other groups of workers could benefit from taking "salt tablets"?

_____

_____

_____

INVESTIGATION 7 　 What are the main symptoms of dehydration?

Terminology

Define each of these terms from the text.

Hydration: _____

Dehydration: _____

TEXT OUTLINE SUMMARY

7.4　What disorders are related to fluid and electrolyte imbalances?

　　7.4.1　Dehydration

　　7.4.2　Heatstroke

　　7.4.3　Water intoxication

Study Questions

Answer these questions to develop the solution to the investigation.

Water output that is greater than water intake can lead to _____.

Excessive water loss commonly results from _____ exercise or

exposure to _____ environmental temperatures.

What are two reasons elderly individuals are more likely to become dehydrated?

_____ and _____

With as little as _____% loss of body weight due to water loss, symptoms of

dehydration will often begin to occur.

What is the first sign of dehydration? _____

Completion Exercise

Use Table 7.6 from the text to complete the following chart.

Using your own weight, determine the amount of fluid weight loss that would lead to symptoms in each column. Your weight is _____ pounds.

Your Weight	1–2% loss	3–5% loss	6–8% loss	9–11% loss

Critical Thinking

If you were stranded at sea aboard a boat with no power, what steps would you take to delay the onset of dehydration?

_____

_____

_____

INVESTIGATION 8   What is hypertension and what lifestyle practices can help to reduce hypertension?

Terminology

Define this term from the text.

Hypertension: _____

TEXT OUTLINE SUMMARY

    7.4.4   Hypertension

        7.4.4.1   What causes hypertension?

        7.4.4.2   What can be done to reduce hypertension?

    7.4.5   Neuropsychiatric disorders

    7.4.6   Muscle disorders

Study Questions

Answer these questions to develop the solution to the investigation.

What is the common name for hypertension? _____

What percent of adults in the United States are affected? _____ What percent

of adults over 65? _____

Name the common symptoms of hypertension. _____

_____

List three medical conditions that occur with increased frequency in persons with hyper-

tension. _____, _____, and _____

What should a normal blood pressure read? _____/_____

Completion Exercise

Complete the following chart and indicate which lifestyle changes should be increased or decreased to have a beneficial/preventive impact on hypertension.

Lifestyle Factor	Decrease	Increase
Salt consumption		
Smoking		
Alcohol consumption		
Weight		
Fruit and vegetable consumption		
Low-fat protein consumption		
Whole-grain consumption		
Exercise		

Critical Thinking

Hypertension is generally a preventable illness. Agree or disagree with this statement and defend your answer with scientific, nutritional facts.

_____

_____

_____

Chapter 8

Nutrients Involved in Antioxidant Function

INVESTIGATION 1 What are free radicals and how can they damage our cells?

Terminology

Define each of these terms from the text.

Atom: _____

Molecule: _____

Oxidation: _____

Reduction: _____

Free radical: _____

TEXT OUTLINE SUMMARY

8.1   What are antioxidants and how does our body use them?

    8.1.1   Oxidation is a chemical reaction in which atoms lose electrons.

        8.1.1.1   Molecules are composed of atoms.

        8.1.1.2   Atoms are composed of particles.

        8.1.1.3   During metabolism, atoms exchange electrons.

    8.1.2   Oxidation sometimes results in the formation of free radicals.

        8.1.2.1   Energy metabolism involves oxidation and gives rise to free radicals.

        8.1.2.2   Other factors can also cause free radical formation.

    8.1.3   Free radicals can destabilize other molecules and damage our cells.

Study Questions

Answer these questions to develop the solution to the investigation.

The smallest physical unit of an element or a compound is called a(n) _____.

A molecule with two or more identical atoms is called a(n) _____.

A molecule with two or more different atoms is called a(n) _____.

During _____ an atom loses an electron.

During _____ an atom gains an electron.

Sometimes during metabolic reactions in the body, an oxygen molecule gains one extra

unpaired _____. The resulting unstable molecule is called a(n)

_____ _____. Unstable free radical molecules attract a(n)

_____ from a nearby stable molecule, thus causing it to become a free radi-

cal and starting a chain reaction of free radical development.

If a free radical occurs in a cell membrane, _____ molecules can be dam-

aged, thus disrupting the integrity of the cell membrane and the cell's function.

Completion Exercise

Label this diagram showing free radical development.

Critical Thinking

Predict what might happen to any tissue or organ that begins unfettered, free radical
development.

_____

_____

_____

INVESTIGATION 2   How do antioxidants protect our cells against oxidative damage from free radicals?

Terminology

Define each of these terms from the text.

Antioxidant: _____

Cofactor: _____

Enzyme: _____

Hydrogen peroxide (H_2O_2): _____

TEXT OUTLINE SUMMARY

8.1.4   Antioxidants work by stabilizing free radicals or opposing oxidation.

Study Questions

Answer these questions to develop the solution to the investigation.

What occurs to free radicals in the presence of antioxidants? _____

What three general groups of compounds exhibit antioxidant function in the body?

_____, _____, and _____

Completion Exercise

Complete the following chart by indicating the correct antioxidant for each explanation.

Compound	Explanation of Most Common Antioxidant Function
	Donates an e⁻ or hydrogen molecule to stabilize free radicals
	Activates antioxidant enzymes
	Converts free radicals to hydrogen peroxide or breaks down hydrogen peroxide to water and oxygen
	Stabilize free radicals, preventing cell and tissue damage

Critical Thinking

Why is H_2O_2 (hydrogen peroxide) used on skin wounds and how is it beneficial?

_____

_____

_____

INVESTIGATION 3   What are some common vitamins and minerals that act as antioxidants in our bodies?

Terminology

Define this term from the text.

Vitamin: _____

TEXT OUTLINE SUMMARY

8.2   A profile of nutrients that function as antioxidants

    8.2.1   Vitamin E

        8.2.1.1   Functions of vitamin E

        8.2.1.2   How much vitamin E should we consume?

            8.2.1.2.1   Recommended dietary allowance for vitamin E

            8.2.1.2.2   Good food sources of vitamin E

        8.2.1.3   What happens if we consume too much vitamin E?

        8.2.1.4   What happens if we don't consume enough vitamin E?

    8.2.2   Vitamin C

        8.2.2.1   Functions of vitamin C

        8.2.2.2   How much vitamin C should we consume?

            8.2.2.2.1   Recommended dietary allowance for vitamin C

            8.2.2.2.2   Good food sources of vitamin C

        8.2.2.3   What happens if we consume too much vitamin C?

        8.2.2.4   What happens if we don't consume enough vitamin C?

    8.2.3   Beta-carotene

        8.2.3.1   Functions of beta-carotene

        8.2.3.2   How much beta-carotene should we consume?

            8.2.3.2.1   Recommended dietary allowance for beta-carotene

            8.2.3.2.2   Good food sources of beta-carotene

        8.2.3.3   What happens if we consume too much beta-carotene?

        8.2.3.4   What happens if we don't consume enough beta-carotene?

    8.2.4   Vitamin A

        8.2.4.1   Functions of vitamin A

            8.2.4.1.1   Vitamin A acts as an antioxidant.

            8.2.4.1.2   Vitamin A is essential to sight.

            8.2.4.1.3   Vitamin A contributes to cell differentiation.

            8.2.4.1.4   Other functions of vitamin A

        8.2.4.2   How much vitamin A should we consume?

            8.2.4.2.1   Recommended dietary intake for vitamin A

            8.2.4.2.2   Good food sources of vitamin A

        8.2.4.3   What happens if we consume too much vitamin A?

        8.2.4.4   What happens if we don't consume enough vitamin A?

Study Questions

Answer these questions to develop the solution to the investigation.

What is the most common fat-soluble vitamin antioxidant? _____

Name the fat-soluble vitamin antioxidant that is necessary for normal vision._____

What is the fat-soluble precursor of vitamin A?_____

The most common water-soluble antioxidant vitamin is _____ .

The mineral antioxidant that is reliably found in organ meats is _____ .

Completion Exercise

Complete the following chart by indicating the correct vitamin and several good dietary sources based on the antioxidant function descriptions.

Antioxidant Function	Vitamin	Good Dietary Sources
Protects fatty tissues and cell membranes; prevents oxidation of LDLs and enhances immunity		
Vitamin A precursor; protects skin and eyes from UV		
Normal vision, fertility, bone growth		
Strong blood vessels and normal healing; enhances immunity and iron absorption		
General immune function and prevents vitamin E oxidation		

Critical Thinking

Discuss the potential impact of a high-protein diet on dietary antioxidant supply.

_____

_____

_____

INVESTIGATION 4   What are the main enzyme systems that minimize oxidative damage?

TEXT OUTLINE SUMMARY

8.2.6   Copper, iron, zinc, and manganese play a peripheral role in antioxidant function.

Study Questions

Answer these questions to develop the solution to the investigation.

How are minerals related to enzymes? _____

What enzyme system converts free radicals to less damaging substances such as hydrogen peroxide? _____

What minerals are necessary cofactors for SOD? _____, _____,

and _____

_____ removes hydrogen peroxide from the body and requires the

mineral _____ to function normally as an antioxidant.

How is hydrogen peroxide removed from the body? _____

Critical Thinking

Enzymes function maximally within a very narrow temperature range in the body. Predict how fever might affect the rate of free radical development and explain why.

_____

_____

_____

INVESTIGATION 5   What are some good food sources of antioxidant nutrients?

TEXT OUTLINE SUMMARY

See Text Outline Summary in Investigation 3 above.

Study Questions

Answer these questions to develop the solution to the investigation.

What are the best dietary sources of antioxidants? _____

What effect does cooking and/or processing have on antioxidants? _____

_____

What animal products have the highest levels of antioxidants? _____

What foods contain the lowest levels of antioxidants? _____

Critical Thinking

Cattle can be fed dried grains and plant products or can be range fed on live grasses. How do you suppose each of these diets would impact the final antioxidant levels in the meat products produced by each feeding method?

_____

_____

_____

INVESTIGATION 6   How are antioxidant nutrients and our potential risk for cancer related?

Terminology

Define each of these terms from the text.

Cancer: _____

Tumor: _____

Malignant: _____

Benign: _____

Carcinogen: _____

TEXT OUTLINE SUMMARY

8.3   What disorders are related to oxidation?

    8.3.1   Cancer

        8.3.1.1   Genetics, lifestyle, and environmental factors can increase our risk for cancer.

            8.3.1.1.1   Tobacco use

            8.3.1.1.2   Sun exposure

            8.3.1.1.3   Nutrition

            8.3.1.1.4   Environmental and occupational exposures

            8.3.1.1.5   Level of physical activity

        8.3.1.2   Antioxidants play a role in preventing cancer.

Study Questions

Answer these questions to develop the solution to the investigation.

What initiates cancer? _____

Free radicals can be powerful carcinogens that can cause damage or mutation to a cell's

_____ .

Cancer arises from a normal cell that has become _____ .

One way to decrease the incidence of cell damage in the body is to decrease the number of circulating _____ _____ .

A diet high in _____-containing fresh fruits and vegetables can be effective in decreasing the number of free radicals in the body.

Increased _____ consumption leads to _____ cancer risk. In addition to minimizing free radical formation and damage, antioxidants are also powerful _____ system stimulants. The immune system plays an important role in the destruction and removal of precancerous abnormal cells from our bodies.

Critical Thinking

What role should antioxidant dietary supplements play with regard to overall general health and specifically with regard to cancer prevention?

_____

_____

_____

What dietary recommendation would you make for someone with cancer and why?

_____

_____

_____

What makes smoking so dangerous?

_____

_____

_____

INVESTIGATION 7   How are phytochemicals related to our potential risk for cancer?

Terminology

Define this term from the text.

Phytochemicals: _____

TEXT OUTLINE SUMMARY

8.3.1.3   Phytochemicals contribute to cancer prevention.

Study Questions

Answer these questions to develop the solution to the investigation.

All phytochemicals are found in _____.

Name the most common phytochemicals: _____

_____

In the laboratory, phytochemicals exhibit clear _____ prevention properties.

It appears that _____ dietary consumption of phytochemicals would tend

to _____ cancer risk.

Completion Exercise

Use Table 8.4 to choose your favorite three food sources for each of the listed phytochemicals.

Phytochemicals	Favorite Three Foods for Providing the Phytochemicals at Left		
Carotenoids			
Organosulfur compounds			
Polyphenols			
Phytoestrogens			

INVESTIGATION 8   How can increasing our intake of antioxidant nutrients reduce our risk for cardiovascular disease?

Terminology

Define this term from the text.

Cardiovascular disease: _____

TEXT OUTLINE SUMMARY

8.3.2   Cardiovascular disease

8.3.3   Vision impairment and other results of aging

Study Questions

Answer these questions to develop the solution to the investigation.

What are the major risk factors for CVD? _____

_____

A recently identified CVD risk factor is low-grade _____, which can cause

damage inside our arteries.

Antioxidants can _____ damage to our arteries and help them to heal if they are damaged.

Low-grade inflammation can be reversed by increasing dietary _____.

Vitamin _____ has been shown to decrease blood clot formation.

Several large surveys have shown that individuals who consume a diet containing many servings of _____ and _____ have a significantly _____ risk of CVD.

Critical Thinking

Based on the information provided in this chapter, do you believe that cardiovascular disease is generally preventable? Explain the reasoning behind your answer.

_____

_____

_____

Chapter 9

Nutrients Involved in Bone Health

INVESTIGATION 1   How are cortical bone and trabecular bone different?

Terminology

Define each of these terms from the text.

Collagen: _____

Cortical bone: _____

Trabecular bone: _____

TEXT OUTLINE SUMMARY

9.1   How does our body maintain bone health?

    9.1.1   Bone composition and structure provide strength and flexibility.

Study Questions

Answer these questions to develop the solution to the investigation.

Bone is made up of approximately _____ % minerals (mostly calcium and

phosphorus) and _____% organic substances (like collagen).

Minerals contribute to a bone's _____, while organic substances contribute

to the bone's _____.

Bone strength and flexibility are also affected by the microscopic _____ of

the bone.

Compact bone is another name for _____, bone which makes up nearly

_____% of the skeleton.

Spongy or cancellous bone is another name for _____ bone, which makes

up only about _____% of our skeleton. _____ bone is found

mostly at the ends of long bones, within the vertebrae, and inside various flat bones of the

skeleton.

Completion Exercise

Complete this chart comparing cortical and trabecular bone.

Type	Percent of Skeleton	Relative Density	Primary Locations in the Skeleton	Relative Turnover Rate	Relative Ability to Detect Bone Loss
Cortical					
Trabecular					

Critical Thinking

It is easier to detect bone loss in trabecular bone than in cortical bone. Why do you think this is so?

_____

_____

_____

INVESTIGATION 2   What are bone growth, bone modeling, and bone remodeling?

Terminology

Define each of these terms from the text.

Bone density: _____

Growth: _____

Modeling: _____

Remodeling: _____

Osteoblasts: _____

Osteoclasts: _____

TEXT OUTLINE SUMMARY

     9.1.2   The constant activity of bone tissue promotes bone health.

          9.1.2.1   Bone growth and modeling determine the size and shape of our bones.

          9.1.2.2   Bone remodeling maintains a balance between breakdown and repair.

Study Questions

Answer these questions to develop the solution to the investigation.

What two processes begin during fetal development in the uterus?

_____ and _____

Which process determines bone size? _____

Which process determines bone shape? _____

Which process directly determines bone density? _____

_____ osteoclast activity results in _____ bone density.

_____ osteoblast activity results in _____ bone density.

Completion Exercise

Place bone growth, bone modeling, *and* bone remodeling *in the correct block in the chart below.*

	Determines bone size
	Begins during fetal development
	Continues into early adulthood
	Primarily an osteoblastic activity
	Determines bone shape
	Begins during fetal development
	Continues into early adulthood
	Primarily an osteoblastic activity
	Maintains integrity of the bone
	Replaces old bone with new bone to maintain mineral balance
	Involves bone resorption and formation
	Occurs predominantly during adulthood
	Both an osteoblastic and osteoclastic activity

Critical Thinking

In what ways would you predict that inadequate dietary calcium intake would affect bone growth, bone modeling, and bone remodeling?

_____

_____

_____

INVESTIGATION 3   What are the most common ways to measure bone density?

Terminology

Define each of these terms from the text.

DEXA: _____

T-score: _____

pDEXA: _____

TEXT OUTLINE SUMMARY

9.2   How do we assess bone health?

    9.2.1   Dual energy x-ray absorptiometry provides a measure of bone density.

    9.2.2   Other bone density measurement tools

Study Questions

Answer these questions to develop the solution to the investigation.

What is the most accurate test for measuring bone density? _____

The level of radiation exposure for this test is less than for a routine _____

x-ray.

Who should have this test done? _____ and younger men and women

who have significant _____ _____ for osteoporosis.

The 'p' in pDEXA stands for what? _____

The pDEXA test x-rays what body part? _____ or _____

Completion Exercise

Complete the following table indicating the meaning and significance of T-scores.

T-score Value	Meaning and Significance of This T-score Range
$-1 \rightarrow +1$	
$-2.5 \rightarrow -1$	
< -2.5	

Critical Thinking

A 65-year-old woman who has regularly drunk about 1 quart of milk daily throughout her life has a T-score of 3.5. The test is repeated and is NOT a mistake. How do you explain what is happening to the bones of this individual?

_____

_____

_____

INVESTIGATION 4   What vitamins and minerals are most important for bone health?

Terminology

Define each of these terms from the text.

Hypercalcemia: _____

Hypocalcemia: _____

Calcitrol: _____

Osteomalacia: _____

Coenzyme: _____

Cofactor: _____

TEXT OUTLINE SUMMARY

9.3   A profile of nutrients that maintain bone health

    9.3.1   Calcium

        9.3.1.1   Functions of calcium

        9.3.1.2   How much calcium should we consume?

            9.3.1.2.1   Recommended dietary intake for calcium

            9.3.1.2.2   Good food sources of calcium

        9.3.1.3   What happens if we consume too much calcium?

        9.3.1.4   What happens if we don't consume enough calcium?

    9.3.2   Vitamin D

        9.3.2.1   Functions of vitamin D

        9.3.2.2   How much vitamin D should we consume?

            9.3.2.2.1   Recommended dietary intake for vitamin D

            9.3.2.2.2   Good food sources of vitamin D

        9.3.2.3   What happens if we consume too much vitamin D?

        9.3.2.4   What happens if we don't consume enough vitamin D?

    9.3.3   Vitamin K

        9.3.3.1   Functions of vitamin K

        9.3.3.2   How much vitamin K should we consume?

            9.3.3.2.1   Recommended dietary intake for vitamin K

            9.3.3.2.2   Good food sources of vitamin K

        9.3.3.3   What happens if we consume too much vitamin K?

        9.3.3.4   What happens if we don't consume enough vitamin K?

Study Questions

Answer these questions to develop the solution to the investigation.

What is the most recognized nutrient with regard to bone health? _____

What is the most abundant *major* mineral in our bodies? _____

Calcium makes up about _____% of our total body weight, and about _____ % of it is in our bones.

In addition to bone strength, we also need adequate levels of calcium in our bodies for what other functions? _____

_____

_____

What other minerals are needed to maintain bone health? _____,

_____, and _____

What two vitamins are necessary in adequate supply for bone health? _____ and _____

Completion Exercise

Complete the following table, indicating the necessary nutrients for maintaining maximal bone health.

	Nutrient	Main Function in Bone Health	Two Good Sources	
Vitamins		Calcium utilization		
		Bone metabolism		
Major minerals		Main component		
		Hydroxyapatite		
		Bone growth		
Trace minerals		New bone growth		

Critical Thinking

What is the most important vitamin necessary to maintain bone health and what groups of people are likely to be deficient in this vitamin? How could this deficiency be resolved?

_____

_____

_____

INVESTIGATION 5   What foods are good sources of dietary calcium?

Terminology

Define the following term from the text.

Bioavailability: _____

TEXT OUTLINE SUMMARY

See the Text Outline Summary for Investigation 4 section 9.3.1.2.2 Good food sources of calcium.

Study Questions

Answer these questions to develop the solution to the investigation.

What are the most common sources of calcium in the United States? _____

Dark green leafy vegetables are a(n) _____ source of bioavailable calcium.

The bioavailability of calcium from spinach is decreased because of the presence of

_____ .

Critical Thinking

If dairy products are a good source of calcium and cows get most of their calcium from grass, what can you predict about the calcium levels in other green leafy foods (since humans don't eat grass)?

_____

_____

_____

Why is it necessary to have knowledge of a variety of good sources of dietary calcium?

_____

_____

_____

INVESTIGATION 6   How can soft drinks be harmful to bone health?

TEXT OUTLINE SUMMARY

See the Text Outline Summary for Investigation 4 section 9.3.4.2.2 Good food sources of phosphorus.

Study Questions

Answer these questions to develop the solution to the investigation.

Phosphorus occurs in many soft drinks (sodas) in what form? _____

Individuals who frequently drink soft drinks are likely to drink less _____

and thus may have an inadequate _____ intake.

Consuming large amounts of acid (such as phosphoric acid in soft drinks) pulls

_____ out of the bones into the blood to neutralize the acid.

Many soft drinks also contain _____, which increases calcium loss

from the body into the urine.

Critical Thinking

The accidental bone fracture rate among teenage girls has been steadily increasing over the past decade in the United States. Discuss the factors that you think may be contributing to this problem.

_____

_____

_____

If the above trend continues, what do you predict will happen to the age of osteoporosis onset in these women?

_____

_____

_____

How can you change your dietary drinking habits in a way to enhance your bone health in the long term?

_____

_____

_____

INVESTIGATION 7   What is osteoporosis and what is its significance to bone health?

Terminology

Define this term from the text.

Osteoporosis: _____

TEXT OUTLINE SUMMARY

9.4   What disorders can result from poor bone health?

    9.4.1   Osteoporosis

Study Questions

Answer these questions to develop the solution to the investigation.

Why is a person with osteoporosis more at risk for bone fractures? _____

_____

What type of bone is most often affected by osteoporosis? _____

Osteoporosis is the single most common cause for hip and spine fractures in what group?

_____

Critical Thinking

Many elderly people "fall and break a hip" every year in the United States. This is usually NOT what occurs. Speculate as to what actually occurs and why.

_____

_____

_____

INVESTIGATION 8 What are the most common risk factors for osteoporosis?

Terminology

Define this term from the text.

Anti-resorptive: _____

TEXT OUTLINE SUMMARY

        9.4.1.1   The impact of aging on osteoporosis risk

        9.4.1.2   Gender and genetics affect osteoporosis risk.

        9.4.1.3   Smoking and poor nutrition increase osteoporosis risk.

        9.4.1.4   The impact of physical activity on osteoporosis risk

        9.1.1.5   Treatments for osteoporosis

    9.4.2   Other bone health disorders

        9.4.2.1   Paget's disease

        9.4.2.2   Osteogenesis imperfecta

Study Questions

Answer these questions to develop the solution to the investigation.

Why are women at greater risk for developing osteoporosis? _____

How does smoking affect bone density? _____

Magnesium, vitamin C, and vitamin K are found in abundance in fresh _____

and _____, which should be consumed daily in the diet.

The best non-drug treatments or preventives for osteoporosis include consuming adequate _____ (a mineral) and vitamin _____, as well as getting

adequate daily _____.

Aside from the impact of adequate nutrition on bone density, what is the most important

factor in preventing osteoporosis? _____

Drugs (anti-resorptives) used to treat osteoporosis generally work in what ways?

_____ and _____

Completion Exercise

If you were at risk for osteoporosis and decided to modify the risk factors that you can impact, rank the modifiable osteoporosis risk factors from easiest to modify to most difficult for you to modify.

_____ smoking

_____ low sun exposure

_____ testosterone deficiency

_____ estrogen deficiency

_____ sedentary lifestyle

_____ body weight

_____ alcohol abuse

_____ repeated falls

_____ low calcium intake

_____ amenorrhea from inadequate nutrition

Critical Thinking

Often when an active person retires, he or she feels it is time for a well-earned rest period in life and often spends hours on the couch in front of a television. Why is that a bad idea?

_____

_____

_____

Chapter 10

Nutrients Involved in Energy Metabolism and Blood Health

INVESTIGATION 1   How do coenzymes enhance the activity of enzymes?

Terminology

Define each of these terms from the text.

Enzyme: _____

Coenzyme: _____

TEXT OUTLINE SUMMARY

10.1   How do our bodies regulate energy metabolism?

      10.1.1   Our bodies require vitamins and minerals to produce energy.

      10.1.2   Some micronutrients assist with nutrient transport and hormone production.

Study Questions

Answer these questions to develop the solution to the investigation.

Why do enzymes need coenzymes to function? _____

Both _____ and _____

are needed together for the body to efficiently release the energy found in the molecules

absorbed into the blood after digestion.

Critical Thinking

Why might some people feel like they have more energy after taking vitamins?

_____

_____

_____

INVESTIGATION 2 What are the B-complex vitamins and how is each one of them involved in energy metabolism?

Terminology

Define each of these terms from the text.

Energy: _____

Metabolism: _____

Text Outline Summary

10.2   A profile of nutrients involved in energy metabolism

    10.2.1   B-complex vitamins act as coenzymes in energy metabolism.

        10.2.1.1   Thiamin (Vitamin B_1)

        10.2.1.2   Riboflavin (Vitamin B_2)

        10.2.1.3   Niacin

        10.2.1.4   Vitamin B_6 (Pyridoxine)

        10.2.1.5   Folate

        10.2.1.6   Vitamin B_{12} (Cobalamin)

        10.2.1.7   Pantothenic acid

        10.2.1.8   Biotin

Study Questions

Answer these questions to develop the solution to the investigation.

The main function of B-complex vitamins in the body is to act as _____ to enzymes that are necessary for the function of energy metabolic pathways; therefore the B-complex vitamins _____ the efficiency of the energy metabolic pathways.

Completion Exercise

Use the main text to find the information necessary to complete the blanks in the following chart. Place an 'x' in the correct corresponding Energy Metabolism columns.

B Vitamin Number/Name	Also Known As:	Energy Metabolism		
		Carbohydrate	Amino Acid	Fat
B_1	thiamine			
B_2	riboflavin			
	niacin			
B_6	pyridoxine			
	folate (folic acid)			
B_{12}	cobalamin			
	pantothenic acid			
	biotin			

Critical Thinking

Is it a good idea for the average person to take a B-complex vitamin supplement daily? Explain your reasoning.

_____

_____

_____

INVESTIGATION 3   What are the most common deficiency disorders for individual B-complex vitamins?

Terminology

Define each of these terms from the text.

Beriberi: _____

Ariboflavinosis: _____

Pellagra: _____

Homocysteine: _____

Atrophic gastritis: _____

10.2.1.9   Consuming adequate B-complex vitamins is easy for most people.

Study Questions

Answer these questions to develop the solution to the investigation.

Inadequate _____ can result in beriberi.

Ariboflavinosis is caused by inadequate _____.

Too little dietary niacin can result in _____.

Adequate folate intake is especially critical during _____ . If it is inadequate during this period, _____ _____ _____ can occur in the newborn.

Inadequate B_{12} can result in _____ anemia.

Completion Exercise

Using the content in Chapter 10 and Table 10.1 in the main text, complete the following chart comparing the B-complex vitamins.

B Vitamin Number/Name	Also Known As:	Deficiency Condition	Good Food Sources
B_1			
B_2			Dairy products, meats, dark green vegetables, enriched cereal, enriched bread
B_6	pyridoxine	no specific one	
		microcytic anemia	
B_{12}		atrophic gastritis	

Critical Thinking

Assuming the typical American diet is heavy on processed foods, what conditions might occur frequently in the United States today if the B-complex vitamins had not been discovered?

_____

_____

_____

INVESTIGATION 4   What are the two most common minerals that function as coenzymes in energy metabolism?

Terminology

Define each of these terms from the text.

Acetylcholine: _____

Goiter: _____

Cretinism: _____

TEXT OUTLINE SUMMARY

10.2.2   Choline

10.2.3   Iodine

10.2.4   Chromium

10.2.5   Manganese

10.2.6   Sulfur

Study Questions

Answer these questions to develop the solution to the investigation.

Chromium plays an important role as a coenzyme in _____ metabolism by enhancing the ability of _____ to facilitate glucose moving from the blood into the cells.

Manganese is a coenzyme involved in _____ _____ and in the formation of urea, a component of urine.

INVESTIGATION 5   What are the four main components of blood?

Terminology

Define each of these terms from the text.

Erythrocytes: _____

Leukocytes: _____

Platelets: _____

Plasma: _____

TEXT OUTLINE SUMMARY

10.3   What is the role of blood in maintaining health?

10.4   A profile of nutrients that maintain health blood

Study Questions

Answer these questions to develop the solution to the investigation.

What are the two kinds of blood cells called? _____ and _____

Which blood component consists of cell fragments? _____

Which blood component is critical in preventing or destroying infection? _____

Which blood cells carry oxygen and carbon dioxide? _____

Completion Exercise

Label the tube of centrifuged blood with the proper location of each of the four main blood components.

Critical Thinking

The HIV virus destroys leukocytes. How does the destruction of leukocytes affect an HIV-infected person's overall health?

_____

_____

_____

If a person is "low" in all of the blood components, what do you suspect has happened or is happening to that person?

_____

_____

_____

INVESTIGATION 6   What role does iron play in oxygen transport?

Terminology

Define each of these terms from the text.

Hemoglobin: _____

Heme: _____

Myoglobin: _____

TEXT OUTLINE SUMMARY

- 10.4.2   Iron
  - 10.4.2.1   Functions of iron
  - 10.4.2.2   How much iron should we consume?
    - 10.4.2.2.1   Recommended dietary intakes for iron
    - 10.4.2.2.2   Good food sources of iron
  - 10.4.2.3   What happens if we consume too much iron?
  - 10.4.2.4   What happens if we don't consume enough iron?
- 10.4.3   Zinc
  - 10.4.3.1   Functions of zinc
  - 10.4.3.2   How much zinc should we consume?
  - 10.4.3.3   What happens if we consume too much zinc?
  - 10.4.3.4   What happens if we don't consume enough zinc?
- 10.4.4   Copper

Study Questions

Answer these questions to develop the solution to the investigation.

The main mineral in both hemoglobin and myoglobin is _____.

Where is hemoglobin found in the body? _____

Where is myoglobin found in the body? _____

What is the role of iron in both hemoglobin and myoglobin? _____

What vitamin enhances iron absorption from food? _____

What chemical found in legumes, rice, and grains inhibits iron absorption? _____

Cooking food in an iron skillet has what benefit? _____

When is iron particularly harmful for human beings? _____

Who needs more iron, men or women? Why? _____

Critical Thinking

Do you think your body contains more hemoglobin or more myoglobin? Why do you think this?

_____

_____

_____

INVESTIGATION 7   How are folate, vitamin B$_{12}$, and vascular disease related?

Terminology

Define each of these terms from the text.

Homocysteine: _____

Vascular: _____

Cardiovascular: _____

Cerebrovascular: _____

Peripheral vascular: _____

TEXT OUTLINE SUMMARY

10.5   What disorders can result from inadequate intakes of nutrients involved in energy metabolism and blood health?

    10.5.1   Neural tube defects

    10.5.2   Vascular disease and homocysteine

Study Questions

Answer these questions to develop the solution to the investigation.

Inadequate levels of what two vitamins prevent homocysteine from being properly metabolized? _____ and _____

In this situation the homocysteine level in the blood _____.

An elevated homocysteine level in the blood is associated with a(n) _____ risk of vascular disease.

Cardiovascular refers to blood vessels found in the _____.

Cerebrovascular refers to blood vessels found in the _____.

Peripheral vascular refers to blood vessels found in the _____.

Critical Thinking

Do you think that the enrichment of foods with folate and B$_{12}$ should be increased? Explain.

_____

_____

_____

INVESTIGATION 8   What are the three most common forms of anemia and how do they differ?

Terminology

Define each of these terms from the text.

Anemia: _____

Pernicious anemia: _____

Macrocytic anemia: _____

TEXT OUTLINE SUMMARY

10.5.3   Anemia

    10.5.3.1   Iron-deficiency anemia

    10.5.3.2   Pernicious anemia

    10.5.3.3   Macrocytic anemia

Study Questions

Answer these questions to develop the solution to the investigation.

What does the word *anemia* mean literally? _____

What is one of the first symptoms a person with anemia feels? _____

What is an obvious sign of anemia that is often visible to others? _____

Completion Exercise

Complete the following table comparing the three common anemias.

Type of Anemia	Size of Erythrocytes	Hemoglobin Amount	Due to Inadequate ...
Iron deficiency			
Pernicious			
Macrocytic			

Critical Thinking

If anemia is not treated, what will be the long-term result? Explain.

_____

_____

_____

Chapter 11

Achieving and Maintaining a Healthful Body Weight

INVESTIGATION 1   What is a healthful weight?

Terminology

Define each of these terms from the text.

Underweight: _____

Overweight: _____

Obesity: _____

Morbid obesity: _____

TEXT OUTLINE SUMMARY

11.1   What is a healthful body weight?

Study Questions

Answer these questions to develop the solution to the investigation.

List some benefits of maintaining a healthful body weight. _____

_____

_____

What is the difference between overweight and obesity? _____

_____

Completion Exercise

In the table below showing the range of possible body weights in order from lightest to heaviest, fill in the most common defining characteristic for each category.

Weight Category	Most Common Defining Characteristic of This Category
Underweight	
Healthful weight	
Overweight	
Obese	
Morbidly obese	

Critical Thinking

How would you characterize your own weight and why do you place yourself in this particular category?

_____

_____

_____

How would your health benefit if you were in a different weight category?

_____

_____

_____

INVESTIGATION 2   What are the most common ways of determining your body composition and finding out if you are a healthful weight?

Terminology

Define each of these terms from the text.

Body composition: _____

Lean body mass: _____

BMI: _____

BIA: _____

NIR: _____

TEXT OUTLINE SUMMARY

11.2   How can you evaluate your body weight?

    11.2.1   Determine your body mass index (BMI).

        11.2.1.1   Why is BMI important?

        11.2.1.2   Limitations of BMI

    11.2.2   Measure your body composition

        11.2.2.1   Underwater weighing method

        11.2.2.2   Skinfold measurement

        11.2.2.3   Bioelectrical impedance analysis

        11.2.2.4   Near infrared reactance

        11.2.2.5   Bod Pod

    11.2.3   Assess your fat distribution patterns.

Study Questions

Answer these questions to develop the solution to the investigation.

Body mass index (BMI) compares a person's _____ with his or her

_____ .

An ideal BMI would be between _____ and _____ .

If a BMI is greater than 30, an individual is at significantly increased risk for what three

diseases? _____ , _____ , and _____

In addition to a calculated BMI, what is the next easiest and most economical method for

an individual to check BMI at home? _____

Completion Exercise

Determine your BMI by completing each of the steps in the following table.

Line	Directions	Result	
		Number	Units
1	Your weight in pounds →		Lbs.
2	Line 1 ÷ 2.2 = your weight in Kg →		Kg
3	Your height in inches →		inches
4	Line 3 × 0.0254 = your height in meters →		m
5	Line 4 × line 4 = the square of your height in meters →		m^2
6	Line 2 ÷ line 5 = your BMI →		

Critical Thinking

How does your BMI compare to a healthful weight?

_____

_____

_____

INVESTIGATION 3 What is energy expenditure and how is it related to weight?

Terminology

Define each of these terms from the text.

Apple-shaped fat distribution: _____

Pear-shaped fat distribution: _____

Energy intake: _____

Energy expenditure: _____

BMR: _____

TEXT OUTLINE SUMMARY

11.3   What makes us gain and lose weight?

     11.3.1   We gain or lose weight when our energy intake and expenditure are out of balance.

         11.3.1.1   Energy intake is the food we eat each day.

         11.3.1.2   Energy expenditure includes more than just physical activity.

             11.3.1.2.1   Our basal metabolic rate (BMR) is our energy expenditure at rest.

             11.3.1.2.2   The thermic effect of food is the energy expended to process food.

             11.3.1.2.3   The energy cost of physical activity is highly variable.

Study Questions

Answer these questions to develop the solution to the investigation.

Which fat distribution pattern is associated with increased disease risk? _____

Energy output is another name for what? _____

To maintain energy balance, _____ must be equal to _____.

To gain weight, _____ must be greater than _____.

To lose weight, _____ must be greater than _____.

What is an extremely healthful way to increase your daily energy expenditure (output)?

_____

Your BMR accounts for approximately how much of your daily energy expenditure?

_____%

Completion Exercise

Both energy intake and energy output must be balanced for a person to maintain weight. In the table below, indicate what happens to the dietary intake or the activity level when a person moves from a category in the Initial Weight column to one in the Resulting Weight column.

Initial Weight	Resulting Weight	Dietary Intake	Activity Level (Exercise)
Underweight	Healthful weight	Does not change	
			Does not change
Healthful	Gain	Does not change	
			Does not change
	Maintain	Does not change	
			Does not change
	Lose	Does not change	
			Does not change
Overweight (to any degree)	Gain	Does not change	
			Does not change
	Maintain	Does not change	
			Does not change
	Lose	Does not change	
			Does not change

Critical Thinking

Often people are less active and eat more during holidays and family celebrations. What advice would you give to individuals in this situation to "balance out" their energy and to return them to their pre-holiday or pre-celebration state?

_____

_____

_____

INVESTIGATION 4   What are several genetic theories thought to have a significant influence on weight?

Terminology

Define each of these terms from the text.

Thrifty gene theory: _____

Set point theory: _____

Leptin: _____

TEXT OUTLINE SUMMARY

      11.3.2   Genetic factors affect body weight.

          11.3.2.1   The thrifty gene theory

          11.3.2.2   The set point theory

          11.3.2.3   The leptin theory

Study Questions

Answer these questions to develop the solution to the investigation.

Where is the "thrifty gene" located? _____

Weight that stays within a relatively narrow range and does not fluctuate significantly with changes in eating is the result of the _____ theory. How does this affect potential weight loss? _____

_____

Mice that produce inadequate leptin become _____ .

Critical Thinking

If leptin injections could cause rapid, effective weight loss and these injections were available over the counter, what effect do you think this would have on the obesity problem in the United States?

_____

_____

_____

INVESTIGATION 5   How do childhood experiences affect adult weight and the risk for adult obesity?

TEXT OUTLINE SUMMARY

11.3.3   Childhood weight influences adult weight.

11.3.4   Behavioral factors affect food choices and body weight.

      11.3.4.1   Composition of the diet

      11.3.4.2   Hunger versus appetite

Study Questions

Answer these questions to develop the solution to the investigation.

Behaviors in childhood can become _____ in adulthood.

Children who are sedentary and consume excess fats and sugars are likely to become adults who are _____. This will likely have what effect on the adult weight of this individual? _____

Children who play outside a lot and are quite active are likely to have what activity level as adults? _____

We learn many of our eating patterns and activity level patterns from our

_____.

Critical Thinking

Think about what might happen to a five-year-old, undernourished orphan who was adopted by a well-to-do family (although not well educated in nutrition) who then provided the child with "good" foods like ice cream, milkshakes, hamburgers, hot dogs, French fries, doughnuts, cakes, pies, sweets of all kinds, and soda. Describe what this child might be like at age six.

_____

_____

_____

INVESTIGATION 6   What are some social factors affecting body weight?

TEXT OUTLINE SUMMARY

11.3.5   Social factors influence behavior and body weight.

11.4   How many kilocalories do you need?

11.5   How can you achieve and maintain a healthful body weight?

    11.5.1   Healthful weight change involves moderation and consistency.

    11.5.2   Safe and effective weight loss

        11.5.2.1   Eat smaller portions of lower-fat foods.

        11.5.2.2   Participate in regular physical activity.

        11.5.2.3   Weight loss can be enhanced with prescribed medications.

        11.5.2.4   Using dietary supplements to lose weight is controversial.

    11.5.3   Safe and effective weight gain

        11.5.3.1   Eat more energy than is expended.

        11.5.3.2   Protein supplements do not increase muscle growth or strength.

Study Questions

Answer these questions to develop the solution to the investigation.

List some social factors that have a direct effect on our weight at any age. _____

_____

_____

The presence of vending machines containing junk food tends to have what effect on a

person's consumption of junk food? _____

How does watching television affect an individual's weight? _____

_____

How might "teen magazines" and TV networks such as MTV adversely affect the eating

habits of teens? _____

Critical Thinking

How do you eat differently during particular social events that you participate in?

_____

_____

_____

What social events do you participate in where food is NOT a significant part of the
event?

_____

_____

_____

What are your favorite foods and why do you like them?

_____

_____

_____

When were you first exposed to these favorite foods?

_____

_____

_____

Why do you "hate" the foods you do?

_____

_____

_____

INVESTIGATION 7 What are the main terms used with regard to abnormal weight and how does each one of these conditions adversely affect health?

Terminology

Define each of these terms from the text.

Underweight: _____

Overweight: _____

Obesity: _____

Morbid obesity: _____

TEXT OUTLINE SUMMARY

11.6   What disorders are related to energy intake?

    11.6.1   Underweight

    11.6.2   Overweight

    11.6.3   Obesity and morbid obesity

        11.6.3.1   What causes obesity?

            11.6.3.1.1   Genetic factors

            11.6.3.1.2   Childhood overweight and obesity are linked to adult obesity

Study Questions

Answer these questions to develop the solution to the investigation.

What are some medical problems that can result from being underweight? _____

_____

How does obesity affect overall health? _____

_____

What are the most significant health dangers from morbid obesity? _____

_____

Completion Exercise

Determine your BMR and total daily energy needs by working through the following table.

Line	Directions	Result Number	Units
1	Your weight in pounds →		Lbs.
2	Line 1 divided by 2.2 = your weight in Kg →		Kg
3	Line 2 multiplied by 1 kcal/hour = number of kcal you need for one hour. Note: This number will be the same as line 2, but the units are different. →		kcal/hr
4	Line 3 is now multiplied by 24 hours = total kcal needed per day →		kcal/d
5	If you are a woman, multiply line 4 by 0.9 = your total kcal needed per day →		kcal/d
6	Using the chart on page 21 of this chapter, determine what activity level most closely fits you and enter the average % of that level or the percent within an activity level range that you believe to be most accurate for you. →		% BMR
7	If you are a male, multiply line 4 by line 6 and enter here → If you are a female, multiply line 5 by line 6 and enter here →		Activity kcal/d
8	If you are a male, add line 4 to line 7 for your average daily calorie expenditure. → If you are a female, add line 5 to line 7 for your average daily calorie expenditure. → This is the approximate number of calories you need to take in every day to maintain your current energy balance. →		Average kcal/d needed for energy balance

Critical Thinking

What did you learn about yourself after determining your BMR?

_____

_____

_____

Do your eating habits generally support a positive energy balance or a negative energy balance?

_____

_____

_____

How can you move both your eating habits and your activity level closer to overall balance?

_____

_____

_____

What are your feelings when you see someone who is obese or morbidly obese?

_____

_____

_____

How would you interact with this person?

_____

_____

_____

How would you discuss weight issues versus health with this individual?

_____

_____

_____

INVESTIGATION 8   What are some common methods of treating obesity?

Terminology

Define each of these terms from the text.

Gastric: _____

Gastroplasty: _____

Gastric bypass: _____

Gastric banding: _____

Liposuction: _____

Study Questions

Answer these questions to develop the solution to the investigation.

A person gains weight because his/her _____ exceeds his/her

_____ .

How does gastric surgery result in weight loss? _____

_____

How do weight-loss drugs aid weight loss? _____

Completion Exercise

Complete the following chart indicating what you believe *to be the main benefit and main downside to each weight-loss method indicated.*

Weight Loss Method	Main Benefit	Main Drawback
Low-calorie diet		
Daily workout		
Weight-loss drugs		
Gastric surgery		
Liposuction		

Critical Thinking

If someone who was obese approached you and asked you how he or she could lose weight, how would you suggest that this person proceed? Why?

_____

_____

_____

Chapter 12

Nutrition and Physical Activity: Keys to Good Health

INVESTIGATION 1   How do physical activity, leisure-time activity, exercise, and physical fitness compare with each other?

Terminology

Define each of these terms from the text.

Physical activity: _____

Exercise: _____

TEXT OUTLINE SUMMARY

12.1   Physical activity, exercise, and physical fitness: What's the difference?

Study Questions

Answer these questions to develop the solution to the investigation.

Physical activity involves movement produced by muscles that increases daily

_____ expenditure.

Leisure-time activity includes movement activities _____ related to a

person's occupation.

Exercise is a(n) _____ of leisure-time activity.

Physical fitness arises out of the relationship between _____ and

_____ _____.

The physically fit person carries out daily activities with _____ and

_____.

Completion Exercise

Complete the following chart indicating how you personally could increase each one of the measures of physical fitness.

Physical Fitness Measure	How Could You Increase This Measure?
Cardiorespiratory	
Muscular strength	
Muscular endurance	
Flexibility	

Critical Thinking

What small (but significant) changes can you make in your daily routine to increase your physical activity?

_____

_____

_____

How would an increased level of physical fitness enhance your life?

_____

_____

_____

INVESTIGATION 2   What are the main benefits of regularly engaging in physical activity?

TEXT OUTLINE SUMMARY

12.2   Why engage in physical activity?

Study Questions

Answer these questions to develop the solution to the investigation.

List all of the common medical conditions that are less likely to occur in physically fit individuals. _____

Completion Exercise

For each of the conditions in the table below, indicate the effect that increased physical activity would have on it.

Parameter or Condition	Likely Effect of Increased Physical Activity
sleep	
immune system	
anxiety	
mental stress	
depression	
fatigue from chemotherapy	
pregnancy and delivery	

Critical Thinking

Discuss the benefits of making physical education mandatory from elementary school through high school.

_____

_____

_____

What would be the benefit of making physical education mandatory in college?

_____

_____

_____

INVESTIGATION 3   What are the main components of fitness?

Terminology

Define each of these terms from the text.

Cardiorespiratory: _____

Musculoskeletal: _____

Strength: _____

Endurance: _____

Flexibility: _____

Body composition: _____

See the Text Outline Summary in Investigation 2.

Study Questions

Answer these questions to develop the solution to the investigation.

Fitness of the heart and lungs is called _____ fitness.

Fitness of the muscles and bones is called _____ fitness.

Which subcomponent of musculoskeletal fitness is defined as the maximal tension that can be attained by a muscle contraction? _____

Which subcomponent of musculoskeletal fitness is defined as the ability of muscle to maintain submaximal force for an extended period of time? _____

What is the term describing the ability to maximally move joints? _____

Body fat percentage is a component of _____ _____.

Critical Thinking

What additional indicators of fitness can you add to those already mentioned in the text?

_____

_____

_____

INVESTIGATION 4   What is the FIT principle and how can you calculate your maximal and training range heart rate?

Terminology

Define each of these terms from the text.

Resistance training: _____

Overload principle: _____

Intensity: _____

12.3   What is a sound fitness program?

    12.3.1   A sound fitness program meets your personal goals.

    12.3.2   A sound fitness program is fun.

    12.3.3   A sound fitness program includes variety and consistency.

    12.3.4   A sound fitness program appropriately overloads the body.

        12.3.4.1   Frequency

        12.3.4.2   Intensity

        12.3.4.3   Time of activity

    12.3.5   A sound fitness program includes a warm-up and a cool-down period.

Study Questions

Answer these questions to develop the solution to the investigation.

In the FIT principle, the F stands for _____; the I stands for _____; and the T stands for _____.

Completion Exercise

Complete the following exercise to determine your maximum heart rate and training heart rate.

To determine your maximal heart rate, subtract your age from 220. Enter that number here _____.

Multiply your maximal heart rate by 0.6 to determine the lower number of your training range heart rate: _____. Multiply your maximal heart rate by 0.8 to determine the upper number of your training range heart rate: _____.

Critical Thinking

Is it possible to exercise too much? Explain.

_____

_____

_____

INVESTIGATION 5 What are the main processes that break down fuels in our body to support physical activity?

Terminology

Define each of these terms from the text.

Adenosine triphosphate (ATP): _____

Creatine phosphate (CP): _____

Aerobic: _____

Anaerobic: _____

Glycolysis: _____

Pyruvic acid: _____

Lactic acid: _____

TEXT OUTLINE SUMMARY

12.4 What fuels our activities?

    12.4.1 The ATP-CP energy system uses creatine phosphate to regenerate ATP.

    12.4.2 The breakdown of carbohydrates provides energy for brief and long-term exercise.

    12.4.3 Anaerobic breakdown of fats supports exercise of low intensity and long duration.

    12.4.4 Amino acids are not major sources of fuel during exercise.

Study Questions

Answer these questions to develop the solution to the investigation.

What is the body's energy currency? _____

ATP is generated from the breakdown of _____, _____, and

_____.

The breakdown of carbohydrates, specifically glucose, is called what? _____

Glycolysis in the presence of adequate oxygen (aerobic) produces _____ acid.

Glycolysis without adequate oxygen (anaerobic) produces _____ acid.

Muscle fatigue and soreness come from buildup of _____ acid in the muscles.

Low-intensity, long-duration exercise uses _____ as the primary energy source.

Maximal-intensity exercise uses _____ as the energy source.

Proteins, made of _____ acids, are not normally used as fuel for exercise, but are used for _____ after exercise.

Critical Thinking

To lose weight by decreasing body fat, what type of exercise would you suggest? Why?

_____

_____

_____

INVESTIGATION 6   What are three ways nutrient needs change in response to a significant increase in training or physical activity?

Terminology

Define each of these terms from the text.

Carbohydrate loading: _____

Glycogen: _____

TEXT OUTLINE SUMMARY

12.4.5   Carbohydrate needs increase for many active people.

    12.4.5.1   How much of an athlete's diet should be carbohydrates?

    12.4.5.2   When should carbohydrates be consumed?

    12.4.5.3   What food sources of carbohydrates are good for athletes?

    12.4.5.4   When does carbohydrate loading make sense?

12.4.6   Moderate fat consumption is enough to support most activities.

12.4.7   Active people need more protein than do inactive people, but many already eat enough.

12.4.8   Regular exercise increases our need for fluids.

    12.4.8.1   Functions of water

    12.4.8.2   Cooling mechanisms

    12.4.8.3   Dehydration and heat-related illnesses

        12.4.8.3.1   Heat syncope

        12.4.8.3.1   Heat cramps

        12.4.8.3.1   Heat exhaustion

        12.4.8.3.1   Heatstroke

12.4.9   Inadequate intakes of some vitamins and minerals can diminish health and performance.

    12.4.9.1   B-complex vitamins

    12.4.9.2   Calcium and the female athlete triad

    12.4.9.3   Iron

Study Questions

Answer these questions to develop the solution to the investigation.

Increased physical activity levels generally require increased consumption of

_____ for fuel.

Carbohydrate loading insures maximal supplies of _____ .

Most activities require only _____ levels of dietary fat consumption.

Increased activity levels require sufficient dietary protein to facilitate tissue

_____ after exercise.

Sweating, from increased activity, results in the need for increased _____

intake.

The _____ vitamins are directly involved in energy metabolism and may

need to be taken as a supplement to burn fuel efficiently.

Critical Thinking

Before participating in a competitive athletic event such as a marathon, what recommendations would you give an athlete about eating before the event? Why?

_____

_____

_____

INVESTIGATION 7   What are the four main heat-caused illnesses and how are they different?

Terminology

Define this term from the text.

Evaporative cooling: _____

TEXT OUTLINE SUMMARY

See Text Outline Summary section 12.4.8.3 in Investigation 6.

Study Questions

Answer these questions to develop the solution to the investigation.

Water is essential for maintaining _____ balance and preventing

_____ .

Inadequate water intake can lead to _____ , which can progress to a heat-related illness.

Standing still too long in heat can result in passing out from _____

_____ .

Muscle spasms resulting from dehydration-induced electrolyte imbalance are called

_____ _____ .

A heat illness characterized by excessive sweating is called _____

_____ .

A heat illness characterized by hot, dry skin and elevated body temperature is called

_____ .

Completion Exercise

Complete the following table comparing the characteristics of the four main dehydration-related conditions.

Condition	Dehydration	Muscle Spasms	Sweating
Heat syncope			
Heat cramps		YES	
Heat exhaustion			
Heatstroke			

Critical Thinking

Why is heatstroke the most severe of the heat-caused illnesses?

_____

_____

_____

INVESTIGATION 8   What are some benefits and risks of four widely touted common ergogenic aids?

Terminology

Define each of these terms from the text.

Ergogenic aids: _____

Placebo effect: _____

TEXT OUTLINE SUMMARY

12.5   Are ergogenic aids necessary for active people?

    12.5.1   Anabolic products are touted as muscle and strength enhancers.

        12.5.1.1   Anabolic steroids

        12.5.1.2   Androstenedione and dehydroepiandrosterone (DHEA)

        12.5.1.3   Gamma-hydroxybutyric acid (GHB)

        12.5.1.4   Creatine

    12.5.2   Some products are said to optimize fuel use during exercise.

        12.5.2.1   Caffeine

        12.5.2.2   Ephedrine

        12.5.2.3   Carnitine

        12.5.2.4   Chromium

        12.5.2.5   Ribose

Study Questions

Answer these questions to develop the solution to the investigation.

Testosterone-based drugs that have been used extensively by strength and power athletes are called _____ _____.

Testosterone precursors that are marketed to increase testosterone levels include

_____ and _____.

_____ has been promoted as an alternative to anabolic steroids for building muscle.

_____ supposedly results in increased ATP production.

Completion Exercise

Complete the following table comparing the main benefits and risks of four common ergogenic aids.

Ergogenic Aid	Benefits	Drawbacks/Risks
Anabolic steroids	increase muscle size, strength, and speed	
Testosterone precursors	none	
GHB	none	
Creatine	enhances performance for anaerobic-type events	

Critical Thinking

"A diet containing fresh fruits and vegetables, range-fed meat, and minimally processed foods is the best ergonenic aid." Is this statement accurate or not? Why?

_____

_____

_____

Chapter 13

Disordered Eating

INVESTIGATION 1   How do eating disorders occur on a continuum?

Terminology

Define each of these terms from the text.

Body image: _____

Continuum: _____

TEXT OUTLINE SUMMARY

13.1   Eating behaviors occur on a continuum.

Study Questions

Answer this question to develop the solution to the investigation.

To which factors are eating disorders most often directly related? _____

CRITICAL THINKING

What do you think of your body?

_____

_____

_____

How do you feel about food?

_____

_____

_____

What is the relationship between food and your body that you have created?

_____

_____

_____

INVESTIGATION 2 What is the difference between disordered eating behaviors and true clinical eating disorders?

Terminology

Define each of these terms from the text.

Eating disorder: _____

Disordered eating: _____

TEXT OUTLINE SUMMARY

13.2 What is the difference between an eating disorder and disordered eating?

Study Questions

Answer these questions to develop the solution to the investigation.

_____ are psychiatric illnesses that must be diagnosed by a physician.

The two main eating disorders are _____ and _____.

Disordered eating is _____ on the continuum of eating disorders.

Disordered eating is characterized by _____ or _____

eating patterns used to change body weight.

Critical Thinking

What role do you believe denial might play in eating disorders? Explain.

_____

_____

_____

What role do you believe denial might play in disordered eating? Explain.

_____

_____

_____

INVESTIGATION 3 What factors may contribute to the development of an eating disorder?

Terminology

Define this term from the text.

Sociocultural values: _____

13.3   What factors contribute to the development of eating disorders?

    13.3.1   Family environment

    13.3.2   Unrealistic media images

    13.3.3   Sociocultural values

    13.3.4   Personality traits

    13.3.5   Genetic and biological factors

Study Questions

Answer these questions to develop the solution to the investigation.

Eating and meal rituals, and attitudes toward food related to a specific relative, are determined largely by one's _____ environment.

Teenagers often feel that their bodies are inadequate or unacceptable because of the huge influence of _____ media images.

Peer teasing about weight is an example of how _____ values can impact body image and thus lead to eating disorders.

Patients with _____ nervosa often exhibit personality traits including increased obsessive-compulsive behavior and perfectionism.

Patients with _____ nervosa often exhibit personality traits including impulsiveness, low self-esteem, and behaviors that seek attention and admiration.

Anorexia nervosa or bulimia nervosa is more likely to occur in individuals who have a relative with one of these disorders; this is known as a(n) _____ or biological factor.

Completion Exercise

Think of several individuals you know well who do not have bodies of a healthy weight. Identify specific characteristics you see that might have an influence on their weight. Write the characteristics in the correct boxes in the table below.

Factors Contributing to Eating Disorders	Individual 1	Individual 2
Family environment		
Unrealistic media images		
Sociocultural values		
Personality traits		
Possible genetic or biological factors		

Critical Thinking

What effect does your family environment, both now and when you were younger, have on your eating habits today?

_____

_____

_____

How much do TV and movies affect your feelings about your body?

_____

_____

_____

Do these feelings ever directly or indirectly influence the way you eat?

_____

_____

_____

INVESTIGATION 4   What are the similarities and differences found in anorexia nervosa, bulimia nervosa, binge eating, and chronic dieting?

Terminology

Define each of these terms from the text.

Anorexia nervosa: _____

Amenorrhea: _____

Bulimia nervosa: _____

Binge eating: _____

Purging: _____

Chronic: _____

Chronic dieting: _____

Weight cycling: _____

TEXT OUTLINE SUMMARY

13.4   What does an eating disorder look like?

    13.4.1   Anorexia nervosa is a potentially deadly eating disorder.

        13.4.1.1   Symptoms of anorexia nervosa

        13.4.1.2   Health risks associated with anorexia nervosa

    13.4.2   Bulimia nervosa is characterized by bingeing and purging.

        13.4.2.1   Symptoms of bulimia nervosa

        13.4.2.2   Health risks of bulimia nervosa

13.5   What does disordered eating look like?

    13.5.1   Binge-eating disorder can cause significant weight gain.

        13.5.1.1   Symptoms of binge-eating disorder

        13.5.1.2   Health risks of binge-eating disorder

    13.5.2   Chronic dieting is a common pattern of disordered eating.

        13.5.2.1   Symptoms of chronic dieting

        13.5.2.2   Health risks associated with chronic dieting

Study Questions

Answer these questions to develop the solution to the investigation.

_____ is characterized by an individual who consistently and purposefully maintains a body weight below normal using any means possible.

Amenorrhea or lack of menstrual periods is a characteristic of _____ nervosa.

Bulimia nervosa is characterized by episodes of _____ eating followed by _____ to get the consumed food out of the body as quickly as possible.

A stressful event or experience can often lead to an eating _____ for emotional comfort.

Consistently and successfully restricting food intake to maintain an average or below average body weight is known as _____ dieting.

Completion Exercise

Complete the following table comparing several eating disorders and disordered eating patterns.

	Characteristics	Male/Female Frequency	Symptoms	Health Risks
Anorexia nervosa				
Bulimia nervosa				
Binge eating				
Chronic dieting				

Critical Thinking

What specific eating behaviors might lead you to suspect that someone has an eating disorder?

_____

_____

_____

Who do you think is more likely to "talk" about weight issues, someone with an eating disorder or someone with disordered eating? Explain.

_____

_____

_____

INVESTIGATION 5   How would you discuss an eating disorder with a friend or relative? What steps would you use?

Text Outline Summary

See the Highlight box on p. 471, Discussing an eating disorder with a friend or family member: What do you say?

Critical Thinking

Describe the steps you would use in discussing an eating disorder with someone to whom you are close.

1. _____

2. _____

3. _____

4. _____

5. _____

6. _____

7. _____

INVESTIGATION 6   What is the female athlete triad and what are its three components?

Terminology

Define each of these terms from the text.

Syndrome: _____

Female athlete triad: _____

Osteoporosis: _____

TEXT OUTLINE SUMMARY

13.6   What is the female athlete triad?

    13.6.1   Sports that emphasize leanness increase the risk for the female athlete triad.

    13.6.2   Three disorders characterize the female athlete triad.

        13.6.2.1   Disordered eating

        13.6.2.2   Menstrual dysfunction

        13.6.2.3   Osteoporosis

    13.6.3   Recognizing and treating the female athlete triad can be challenging.

Study Questions

Answer these questions to develop the solution to the investigation.

The female athlete triad is the name of a syndrome consisting of three medical conditions found frequently in female athletes that includes: _____, _____, and _____.

The risk is increased for women who participate in sports that require body

_____.

Osteoporosis is significantly increased in these women as a consequence of the low levels of the hormones _____ and _____ that occur with amenorrhea.

The female athlete triad results when food intake is consistently _____ what is needed to maintain a healthy body.

Critical Thinking

What changes need to be made with regard to the unhealthy and unrealistic weight standards for female athletes? How would you go about making this happen?

_____

_____

_____

INVESTIGATION 7   What treatment options are available for people with anorexia nervosa and bulimia nervosa?

Terminology

Define each of these terms from the text.

Psychosocial: _____

Psychotropic: _____

Antidepressant: _____

TEXT OUTLINE SUMMARY

13.7   What therapies work for people with an eating disorder?

    13.7.1   Choosing a treatment approach for an eating disorder

    13.7.2   Treatment options for patients with anorexia nervosa

        13.7.2.1   Nutritional therapies are critical in anorexia nervosa treatment.

        13.7.2.2   Psychosocial interventions are important.

        13.7.2.3   Psychotropic medications may be helpful.

    13.7.3   Treatment options for patients with bulimia nervosa

        13.7.3.1   Nutritional therapies are critical in bulimia nervosa treatment.

        13.7.3.2   Psychosocial interventions are important.

        13.7.3.3   Antidepressant medications may be helpful.

Study Questions

Answer this question to develop the solution to the investigation.

Treating eating disorders is most successful when a(n) _____ approach is used.

Completion Exercise

Complete the table below, indicating the key factors in each of the main treatment methods for anorexia nervosa and bulimia nervosa.

Disorder	Nutritional Therapy	Psychosocial Interventions	Medications
Anorexia nervosa			psychotropics
Bulimia nervosa			antidepressants

Critical Thinking

What issues could possibly sabotage eating disorder treatment and how might they be prevented?

_____

_____

_____

INVESTIGATION 8 How can eating disorders be prevented?

13.8   How can we prevent eating disorders and disordered eating?

Study Questions

Answer this question to develop the solution to the investigation.

The most obvious way to prevent eating disorders is to preemptively reverse each one of

the _____ of eating disorders.

Critical Thinking

How would you deal with each one of the following factors that contribute to eating disorders in order to reverse its negative impact on someone you are very close to?

Family environment

_____

_____

_____

Unrealistic media images

_____

_____

_____

Sociocultural values

_____

_____

_____

Personality traits

_____

_____

_____

Genetic and biological factors

_____

_____

_____

Chapter 14

Food Safety and Technology: Impact on Consumers

INVESTIGATION 1   Why is food safety such an important concern?

Terminology

Define each of these terms from the text.

Food-borne illness: _____

Processed foods: _____

TEXT OUTLINE SUMMARY

14.1   Why is food safety important?

    14.1.1   Food-borne illness affects seventy-six million Americans each year.

    14.1.2   Spoilage affects a food's appeal and safety.

    14.1.3   Technological manipulation of food raises safety concerns.

    14.1.4   Government regulations control food safety.

Study Questions

Answer these questions to develop the solution to the investigation.

How many Americans are affected with food-borne illness every year? _____

Food starts to break down when it is harvested due to _____, which are

naturally found in the food, and _____ on the surface of the food.

Three factors that contribute to food spoilage are _____,

_____, and _____.

Completion Exercise

Consider the foods that you eat daily and consider how they are processed and/or packaged in ways that prevent spoilage. Oxygen, heat, and light are the three factors that enhance food spoilage. Complete the following table using examples of how the foods you consume frequently are processed or packaged to decrease the effects of oxygen, heat, and light and thus decrease the rate of spoilage.

Oxygen			
Heat			
Light			

Critical Thinking

What do you think is the most important source of wrong information about food handling and preparation?

_____

_____

_____

How significant do you think this "wrong information" is with regard to food-borne illness?

_____

_____

_____

Would it be beneficial to have only one government agency to deal with food safety? Explain.

_____

_____

_____

INVESTIGATION 2   What microorganisms cause food-borne illness?

Terminology

Define each of these terms from the text.

Microbes: _____

Bacteria: _____

Virus: _____

Prion: _____

Helminth: _____

Parasite: _____

Fungus: _____

TEXT OUTLINE SUMMARY

14.2   What causes food-borne illness?

    14.2.1   Food-borne illness is caused by microorganisms and their toxins.

        14.2.1.1   Some microbes release toxins.

    14.2.2   Our bodies respond to food-borne microbes and toxins with acute illness.

    14.2.3   Certain environmental conditions help microbes multiply in foods.

    14.2.4   Food allergies can also cause illness.

Study Questions

Answer these questions to develop the solution to the investigation.

Most food-borne illnesses are caused by _____ in the food, or toxic by-products from _____ .

Illnesses directly caused by microbes in food are called _____ .

A food-borne illness caused by toxins (poisons) secreted by microbes in food is called

_____ .

Toxins that damage the nervous system and often cause paralysis are called

_____ .

Toxins that affect the gastrointestinal system, often by causing severe diarrhea and/or vomiting, are called _____ .

Food _____ can also cause immediate or delayed reactions causing a range of problems from mild itching to death.

Completion Exercise

Complete the table below, giving one example for each category of microbes.

Microbes Causing Food Infection		
Microbe Group	**Name of Specific Microbe**	**Name of Disease**
Bacteria		
Viruses		
Prions		
Helminths		
Fungi		
Microbes Causing Food Intoxication		
Microbe Group	**Name of Specific Microbe**	**Name of Disease**
Bacteria		
Fungi		

Critical Thinking

How many food-borne infections could be prevented by hand-washing? Explain.

_____

_____

_____

INVESTIGATION 3　How can you minimize the risk of food-borne illness at home, when eating out, and when traveling in foreign countries?

Terminology

Define each of these terms from the text.

Cross contamination: _____

Biotoxins: _____

TEXT OUTLINE SUMMARY

14.3　How can you prevent food-borne illness?

    14.3.1　When preparing foods at home

        14.3.1.1　Wash your hands.

        14.3.1.2　Wash kitchen utensils and surfaces.

        14.3.1.3　Isolate raw foods.

        14.3.1.4　Store foods in the refrigerator or freezer.

            14.3.1.4.1　Shopping tips

            14.3.1.4.2　Refrigerating foods

            14.3.1.4.3　Freezing and thawing foods

            14.3.1.4.4　Molds in refrigerated foods

        14.3.1.5　Cook foods thoroughly.

    14.3.2　When eating out

    14.3.3　When traveling to other countries

Study Questions

Answer these questions to develop the solution to the investigation.

Which foods are most commonly associated with food-borne illness? _____

Foods that come from several animals, such as ground beef or sausage, pose a

_____ risk of causing food-borne illnesses.

_____ foods are least likely to cause food-borne illnesses.

_____ _____ results when bacteria (or other microbes) are

spread from one food to another.

Critical Thinking

Immigrants to the United States who travel back to their home country after living in the United States for a year or more often experience severe gastrointestinal problems from the food. Prior to immigrating, these individuals never experienced such problems. Explain why this might be.

_____

_____

_____

INVESTIGATION 4   What are the advantages and disadvantages of common food preservation methods?

Terminology

Define each of these terms from the text.

Pasteurization: _____

Irradiation: _____

Genetic modification: _____

TEXT OUTLINE SUMMARY

14.4   How is food spoilage prevented?

    14.4.1   Tried and true: preserving foods through natural techniques

        14.4.1.1   Salting and sugaring

        14.4.1.2   Drying

        14.4.1.3   Smoking

        14.4.1.4   Cooling

    14.4.2   Better living through chemistry: Synthetic preservative techniques improve food safety.

        14.4.2.1   Industrial canning

        14.4.2.2   Pasteurization

Study Questions

Answer these questions to develop the solution to the investigation.

To survive, most bacteria that spoil food need adequate moisture, a fairly warm

_____, and a good source of food.

Food preservation methods remove or decrease one or more of the _____

for bacterial survival.

Completion Exercise

Compete the following table showing the advantages and disadvantages of each preservation method.

Food Preservation Technique	Advantages	Disadvantages
Sugaring		significant calories, sweetness
Salting		saltiness, very high sodium level
Drying		food properties change, fewer vitamins
Smoking		need to be protected from insects, animals during storage
Cooling		requires "cool" area or power to cool a warm area
Canning		some change in food characteristics
Pasteurization		does not eliminate all microbes
Chemical preservatives		individual sensitivities
Aseptic packaging		more fragile than rigid containers
Irradiation		unpleasant change in taste and smell in some irradiated foods
Genetic modification		unknown effect of long-term consumption

Critical Thinking

Explain how one of the preservation methods above might have been "discovered."

_____

_____

_____

INVESTIGATION 5   What are food preservatives and why are they used?

Terminology

Define each of these terms from the text.

BHA/BHT: _____

Propionic acid: _____

Sulfites: _____

Nitrates: _____

Nitrites: _____

TEXT OUTLINE SUMMARY

14.4.2.3   Addition of preservatives
    14.4.2.3.1   BHA/BHT
    14.4.2.3.2   Propionic acid
    14.4.2.3.3   Sulfites
    14.4.2.3.4   Nitrates and nitrites
    14.4.2.3.5   Aseptic packaging
14.4.2.4   Irradiation
14.4.2.5   Genetic modification

Study Questions

Answer these questions to develop the solution to the investigation.

All preservatives must be listed in what section of a food label? _____

BHA/BHT prevent _____ and _____ in foods from becoming rancid.

What preservative inhibits mold growth? _____

What preservative (formerly used on salad bar foods) prevents browning and is an antioxidant? _____

Why are stored grapes frequently fumigated with sulfur dioxide? _____

The "fresh" pink color of processed meats often comes from what preservative?

_____

Critical Thinking

In general, what effect do food preservatives have on food shopping frequency? Explain.

_____

_____

_____

How do food preservatives affect food safety and potential food-borne illnesses?

_____

_____

_____

INVESTIGATION 6   How safe are food additives and what is the GRAS list?

Terminology

Define each of these terms from the text.

Additive: _____

Natural: _____

Synthetic: _____

Coal tar: _____

GRAS: _____

Residues: _____

POPs: _____

PCPs: _____

Dioxins: _____

TEXT OUTLINE SUMMARY

14.5   What are food additives, and are they safe?

    14.5.1   Additives can enhance a food's taste, appearance, safety, or nutrition.

        14.5.1.1   Additives can be natural or synthetic.

        14.5.1.2   Flavorings

        14.5.1.3   Colorings

        14.5.1.4   Vitamins and other nutrients

    14.5.2   Are food additives safe?

14.6   Do residues harm our food supply?

    14.6.1   Persistent organic pollutants can cause illness.

        14.6.1.1   Mercury and lead are nerve toxins found in the environment.

        14.6.1.2   Texturizers, stabilizers, and emulsifiers

        14.6.1.3   Humectants and desiccants

    14.6.2   Some additives get into our food unintentionally.

14.7   The GRAS list identifies food additives.

    14.7.1   Industrial pollutants also create residues.

    14.7.2   Reducing POPs is a global concern.

Study Questions

Answer these questions to develop the solution to the investigation.

What government agency regulates food additives in the United States? _____

Food additives enhance a food's _____, _____, _____,
or _____.

Why are flavorings often used in foods? _____

Food colorings made from _____ have been found to cause cancer in animals.

Which additive must be indicated on the product packaging because it can cause an allergic reaction in some people? _____

Pollutants are found in _____ levels in all living organisms.

No food additive will be added to the GRAS list if it has been shown to cause
_____ in animals or humans.

Completion Exercise

Describe what each additive type does in food.

Additives	What Do They Do?
flavorings	
texturizers	
stabilizers	
thickeners	
emulsifiers	
food colors	
humectants	
desiccants	
vitamins	
minerals	
preservatives	

Critical Thinking

What foods that you consume contain the most additives? What foods that you consume contain the least?

_____

_____

_____

INVESTIGATION 7   What are the benefits and safety concerns with regard to pesticides and our food supply?

Terminology

Define each of these terms from the text.

Pesticides: _____

Insecticides: _____

Herbicides: _____

Fungicides: _____

TEXT OUTLINE SUMMARY

14.8   Pesticides protect against crop losses.

    14.8.1   Pesticides can be natural or synthetic.

    14.8.2   Pesticides are potential toxins.

    14.8.3   Government regulations control the use of pesticides.

14.9   Growth hormones are injected into cows to increase production of meat and milk.

Study Questions

Answer these questions to develop the solution to the investigation.

The main purpose for using pesticides during food production is to decrease

_____ loss.

_____ are chemicals that use natural methods to reduce crop damage.

One way to minimize pesticide residue consumption is to _____ all fresh
fruits and vegetables.

Acceptable pesticide residue levels in foods are set by which governmental agency?

_____

Critical Thinking

If pesticides were suddenly banned from use for food production, how would this affect
you and your food shopping? Explain.

_____

_____

_____

INVESTIGATION 8   What are organic foods?

Terminology

Define this term from the text.

Organic: _____

TEXT OUTLINE SUMMARY

14.10   Are organic foods more healthful?

    14.10.1   To be labeled organic, foods must meet federal standards.

    14.10.2   The USDA regulates organic farming.

    14.10.3   Organic foods can be more nutritious.

Study Questions

Answer these questions to develop the solution to the investigation.

To be labeled "organic," a food must be raised without the application of

_____ pesticides.

To be labeled "organic," a food must be raised in accordance with standards set by which

federal agency? _____

To have the USDA's organic label, a food must be at least _____% organic.

When are organic farmers permitted to use synthetic insecticides? _____

_____

Critical Thinking

Organic foods are generally more expensive to buy. How does this affect your food purchasing decisions?

_____

_____

_____

How could the cost of organic foods be decreased?

_____

_____

_____

Chapter 15

Nutrition Through the Lifecycle: Pregnancy and the First Year of Life

INVESTIGATION 1 Why is maintaining a nutritious diet important even before pregnancy occurs?

Terminology

Define each of these terms from the text.

Conception: _____

Teratogen: _____

TEXT OUTLINE SUMMARY

15.1   Starting out right: healthful nutrition in pregnancy

   15.1.1   Is nutrition important before conception?

Study Questions

Answer these questions to develop the solution to the investigation.

Some nutritional deficiency-related problems can occur during the first few weeks after

_____, before a woman even knows she is pregnant.

A woman of child-bearing age should always have adequate intake of _____

to prevent fetal neural tube defects.

Drugs and other nonfood substances ingested during pregnancy could all possibly act as

teratogens, resulting in _____ _____.

Improper nutrition in the male can lead to sperm _____.

INVESTIGATION 2   How are the increasing nutrient requirements during pregnancy related to fetal development?

Terminology

Define each of these terms from the text.

Trimester: _____

Zygote: _____

Embryo: _____

Fetus: _____

Spontaneous abortion: _____

Placenta: _____

Umbilical cord: _____

Gestation: _____

TEXT OUTLINE SUMMARY

15.1.2   Why is nutrition important during pregnancy?
15.1.2.1   The first trimester
15.1.2.2   The second trimester
15.1.2.3   The third trimester
15.1.2.4   Impact of nutrition on maturity and birth weight

Study Questions

Answer these questions to develop the solution to the investigation.

The goal of maintaining proper nutrition during pregnancy is to insure adequate nutrients

to support fetal _____ and to prevent nutritional _____

in the mother.

Spontaneous abortion, also known as _____, occurs most often during

the _____ trimester.

What are the two main roles of the placenta with regard to fetal nutrition?

_____ _____

How is the placenta connected to the fetus? _____

Without adequate nutrition a mother is much more likely to deliver a baby that is

_____ (less than 38 weeks gestation) and/or of

_____ _____ _____ (less than

5.5 pounds).

Completion Exercise

In the chart below, indicate the most important fetal development occurring during each of the trimesters.

Trimester	Most Important Development During This Time Period
1st	
2nd	
3rd	

Critical Thinking

During which trimester is the fetus/embryo most susceptible to nutritional deficiencies that can cause birth defects? Explain.

_____

_____

_____

INVESTIGATION 3   What are the acceptable weight gain ranges for each trimester during pregnancy?

TEXT OUTLINE SUMMARY

15.1.3   How much weight should a pregnant woman gain?

Study Questions

Answer these questions to develop the solution to the investigation.

What is the healthy, average amount of weight a woman should gain during pregnancy?

_____

A small and/or thin woman should gain _____ weight, while a large and/or heavy woman should gain _____ weight.

Completion Exercise

Complete the weight gain chart below for three women of varying weights.

Weight Prior to Pregnancy	Lowest Healthy Weight at End of Pregnancy, Just Prior to Delivery	Highest Healthy Weight at End of Pregnancy, Just Prior to Delivery
100 pounds		
150 pounds		
200 pounds		
250 pounds		

Critical Thinking

How do you think abnormal weight gain (both too much and too little) might affect the fetus?

_____

_____

_____

INVESTIGATION 4   How does lactation occur?

Terminology

Define each of these terms from the text.

Lactation: _____

Colostrum: _____

TEXT OUTLINE SUMMARY

See Text Outline Summary section 15.2.1 in Investigation 5.

Study Questions

Answer these questions to develop the solution to the investigation.

Lactation begins in response to _____ changes occurring in late pregnancy.

The hormone directly responsible for milk production in the breast is _____.

The hormone directly responsible for milk let-down is _____.

Lactation continues in response to regular mammary _____.

The milk that is produced in the breast during the first few days of suckling is called

_____.

How does colostrum help to protect the newborn from infection? _____

Critical Thinking

What conditions might prevent a woman from breast-feeding her infant? Explain.

_____

_____

_____

INVESTIGATION 5   How do the nutrient requirements for pregnant and lactating women compare?

Terminology

Define each of these terms from the text.

Neural tube: _____

Anencephaly: _____

Iron deficiency: _____

Amniotic fluid: _____

TEXT OUTLINE SUMMARY

15.1.4   What are a pregnant woman's nutritional needs?

    15.1.4.1   Macronutrient needs of a pregnant woman

        15.1.4.1.1   Energy

        15.1.4.1.2   Protein and carbohydrate

        15.1.4.1.3   Fat

        15.1.4.1.4   Folate

        15.1.4.1.5   Vitamin B_{12}

        15.1.4.1.6   Vitamin C

        15.1.4.1.7   Vitamin A

        15.1.4.1.8   Vitamin D

        15.1.4.1.9   Calcium

        15.1.4.1.10   Iron

        15.1.4.1.11   Zinc

        15.1.4.1.12   Sodium and iodine

    15.1.4.2   Do pregnant women need supplements?

    15.1.4.3   Fluid needs of pregnant women

Study Questions

Answer these questions to develop the solution to the investigation.

Pregnancy requires adequate nutrient intake to support the _____ of the mother's blood volume, and to support _____ of the uterus, placenta, breasts, increasing body fat levels, and the fetus proper.

Foods consumed during pregnancy should be _____ dense.

Breast-feeding women need even _____ energy than pregnant women need.

Completion Exercise

The table below compares the significant nutrient requirements for both pregnant and nursing women. Complete the Why Needed column for each of the listed nutrients.

Parameter	Comparison of Nutrient Requirements		Why Needed
	Pregnant	**Nursing**	
Energy	300 kcal/day above prepregnancy needs during last two trimesters	500 kcal/day above prepregnancy needs	
Protein	10–15 grams/day above prepregnancy needs	15–20 grams/day above prepregnancy needs	
Carbohydrate	at least 100 grams/day	at least 100 grams/day	
Folate	600 μg/day	500 μg/day	
B_{12}	2.6 μg/day	over 2.6 μg/day	
Calcium	1,000 mg/day	1,000 mg/day; teen mothers 1,300 mg/day	
Supplements	omega-3 fatty acids, multivitamin	omega-3 fatty acids, multivitamin	
Fluid needs	extra	one liter more per day than during pregnancy	

Critical Thinking

There appears to be some discrepancy between WIC program utilization and the percentage of low-birth-weight infants born to some participants. How would you improve the birth outcomes in WIC program participants?

_____

_____

_____

INVESTIGATION 6   What are the primary advantages and the most common challenges of breast-feeding?

Terminology

Define each of these terms from the text.

SIDS: _____

Ovulation: _____

TEXT OUTLINE SUMMARY

15.2.3   Getting real about breast-feeding: pros and cons

    15.2.3.1   Advantages of breast-feeding

        15.2.3.1.1   Nutritional quality of breast milk

        15.2.3.1.2   Protection from infections and allergies

        15.2.3.1.3   Physiologic benefits for mother

        15.2.3.1.4   Mother–infant bonding

        15.2.3.1.5   Convenience and cost

    15.2.3.2   Difficulties encountered with breast-feeding

        15.2.3.2.1   Effects of drugs and other substances on breast milk

        15.2.3.2.2   Maternal HIV infection

        15.2.3.2.3   Conflict between breast-feeding and the mother's employment

        15.2.3.2.4   Social concerns

    15.2.3.3   What about bonding for fathers and siblings?

Study Questions

Answer these questions to develop the solution to the investigation.

The nutritional quality of breast milk _____ over time specifically to meet the nutritional needs of the growing infant.

Breast milk offers significant protection from _____ and _____.

Why does a subsequent pregnancy usually not occur while a woman is breast-feeding?

_____

The intimacy of breast-feeding facilitates _____.

Breast-feeding has a significant _____ benefit when compared to formula feeding.

Completion Exercise

Complete the chart below describing possible drawbacks of breast-feeding.

Situation or Condition	Possible Drawbacks to Breast-Feeding
Drugs, caffeine, alcohol, some foods	
Maternal HIV status	
Employment	
Social concerns	

Critical Thinking

If you were to become a parent in the future, would you plan to breastfeed? Why or why not?

_____

_____

_____

INVESTIGATION 7   How do the growth and activity patterns of infants relate to their changing nutrient needs?

TEXT OUTLINE SUMMARY

15.3   Infant nutrition from birth to one year

    15.3.1   Typical infant growth and activity patterns

    15.3.2   Nutrient needs for infants

        15.3.2.1   Macronutrient needs of infants

        15.3.2.2   Micronutrient needs of infants

        15.3.2.3   Do infants need supplements?

        15.3.2.4   Fluid recommendations for infants

        15.3.2.5   What types of formula are available?

        15.3.2.6   When do infants begin to need solid foods?

        15.3.2.7   Lead poisoning

Study Questions

Answer these questions to develop the solution to the investigation.

Babies have a very _____ metabolic rate.

During the first several months after birth, a baby's activities consist mostly of

_____ and _____.

During the first year of life, an infant's weight generally _____ .

Infants should consume _____ kcal/pound of body weight per day.

Why do newborn infants need vitamin K supplementation? _____

Infants need how many ounces of fluid per pound of body weight per day to prevent

dehydration? _____

If an infant is getting adequate fluid intake, how many wet diapers should occur per day?

_____

Completion Exercise

Complete the following table of nutrient needs for an infant.

Nutrient	Percent of Diet	Reason
Fats	40–50	
Proteins	no more than 20	
Carbohydrates	20–30	

Critical Thinking

Would it be beneficial for all mothers to have a copy of a growth chart (similar to the one found in your textbook in Figure 15.11) during the first year of each child's life? Explain.

_____

_____

_____

If a mother of a new baby has only an adult scale available, how can she weigh her baby and monitor its growth?

_____

_____

_____

INVESTIGATION 8 What are some common nutrient-related concerns for infants?

Terminology

Define each of these terms from the text.

Colic: _____

Dental caries: _____

Study Questions

Answer these questions to develop the solution to the investigation.

What is the best way to minimize food allergies in infants? _____

What condition causes the greatest risk for dehydration in infants? _____

Infants must have an adequate intake of _____ to prevent anemia.

What is most likely the underlying cause of dental caries in infants? _____

Poisoning from _____ can lead to severe nervous and other system impairment.

Critical Thinking

What are the main benefits of breast-feeding and what are the main drawbacks of breast-feeding for the mother and for the infant, as you now see it?

Maternal benefit:

_____

_____

_____

Maternal drawback:

_____

_____

_____

Infant benefit:

_____

_____

_____

Infant drawback:

_____

_____

_____

Chapter 16

Nutrition Through the Lifecycle: Childhood to Late Adulthood

INVESTIGATION 1   What are the similarities and differences in the growth and activity patterns of toddlers and preschoolers?

Terminology

Define this term from the text.

EER: _____

TEXT OUTLINE SUMMARY

16.1   Nutrition for toddlers, aged 1–3 years

    16.1.1   Toddler growth and activity patterns

    16.1.2   What are a toddler's nutrient needs?

        16.1.2.1   Energy and macronutrient recommendations for toddlers

        16.1.2.2   Micronutrient recommendations for toddlers

        16.1.2.3   Fluid recommendations for toddlers

        16.1.2.4   Do toddlers need nutritional supplements?

    16.1.3   Encouraging nutritious food choices with toddlers

    16.1.4   Nutrition-related concerns for toddlers

        16.1.4.1   Continued allergy watch

        16.1.4.2   Obesity: a concern now?

        16.1.4.3   Vegetarian families

16.2   Nutrition for preschoolers, aged 4–5 years

    16.2.1   Preschooler growth and activity patterns

    16.2.2   What are a preschooler's nutrient needs?

        16.2.2.1   Energy and macronutrient recommendations for preschoolers

        16.2.2.2   Micronutrient recommendations for preschoolers

        16.2.2.3   Fluid recommendations for preschoolers

    16.2.3   Encouraging nutritious food choices with preschoolers

    16.2.4   Nutrition-related concerns for preschoolers

        16.2.4.1   Obesity watch: encouraging an active lifestyle

        16.2.4.2   Dental caries

Study Questions

Answer these questions to develop the solution to the investigation.

What occurs to the activity level of children as they move from infancy to preschool age?

_____

What happens to the rate of body growth in children as they move from infancy to

preschool age? _____

Completion Exercise

Calculate the EER (estimated energy requirement) for a toddler.

Enter the child's weight in pounds here _____. Divide this number by 2.2 and

enter here _____. This is the child's weight in Kg. Multiply the child's weight

in Kg by 89 and enter the result here _____. Subtract 80 from this number to

determine the kcal/day for this child. Enter your results here. _____

Critical Thinking

Are naps important to toddlers and preschoolers? Explain your reasoning.

_____

_____

_____

INVESTIGATION 2   How do micronutrient needs change as a child matures from school-aged years to adolescence?

Terminology

Define this term from the text.

Adolescence: _____

TEXT OUTLINE SUMMARY

16.3   Nutrition for school-aged children, age 6–13 years.

    16.3.1   School-age growth and activity patterns

    16.3.2   What are a school-aged child's nutrient needs?

        16.3.2.1   Energy and macronutrient recommendations for school-aged children

        16.3.2.2   Micronutrient recommendations for school-aged children

        16.3.2.3   Fluid recommendations for school-aged children

    16.3.3   Encouraging nutritious food choices with school-aged children

    16.3.4   What is the effect of school attendance on nutrition?

    16.3.5   Are school lunches nutritious?

Study Questions

Answer these questions to develop the solution to the investigation.

Micronutrient needs for children increase only _____ over the preschool years.

What are the two main reasons for the increased need for iron and calcium in adolescents?

1. _____

2. _____

What is the main reason adolescent girls need adequate iron intake? _____

Critical Thinking

How might a vegan diet affect an adolescent female? Explain.

_____

_____

_____

Why are adolescents likely to be deficient in necessary micronutrients?

_____

_____

_____

INVESTIGATION 3   What are the three nutrients of greatest concern when feeding a vegan diet to young children?

Terminology

Define each of these terms from the text.

Vegetarian: _____

Vegan: _____

Bioavailable: _____

TEXT OUTLINE SUMMARY

16.1.4.3   Vegetarian families

Study Questions

Answer these questions to develop the solution to the investigation.

Red meat is an excellent source of what kind of iron? _____

Why is dietary heme iron the best source nutritionally? _____

For growing children, dairy products provide the best source of what nutrient? _____

How much vitamin B_{12} can be obtained from plant foods? _____

Completion Exercise

The chart below lists nutrients that are difficult to obtain from a vegan diet. Complete the chart by indicating why each nutrient is important for growing children to consume.

Nutrient	Why Is This Nutrient Critical for the Growing Child?
Iron	
Protein	
Calcium	
Vitamin B_{12}	

Critical Thinking

What food recommendations would you suggest to a vegan family with a toddler? Explain.

_____

_____

_____

INVESTIGATION 4   What is puberty and how does it change body composition?

Terminology

Define each of these terms from the text.

Puberty: _____

Menarche: _____

TEXT OUTLINE SUMMARY

16.4.1   Adolescent growth and activity patterns

Study Questions

Answer these questions to develop the solution to the investigation.

The development of secondary _____ characteristics is one of the main

defining events of puberty. This results in these individuals being _____

able to reproduce.

Puberty is also marked by a significant _____ spurt.

Completion Exercise

Complete the following table comparing the changing body composition of teenage males and females.

Body Characteristic	Males	Females
Height (20–25% increase)		
Weight		
Sexual development		

Critical Thinking

What effects can changing body composition have on adolescent self-esteem?

_____

_____

_____

INVESTIGATION 5   What are some common factors that can lead to obesity?

TEXT OUTLINE SUMMARY

See the Text Outline Summary in Investigation 2 above.

Study Questions

Answer these questions to develop the solution to the investigation.

Obesity is caused in part by eating _____ and moving (exercising)

_____.

Today, the general trend in school-age children is to engage in _____

physical activity than in the preschool years.

Generally, teenagers engage in even _____ physical activity than in

the grade school years.

Completion Exercise

Complete the table below comparing various common situations of children today with regard to food consumption and weight.

Situation	Often Results in What Effect on Food Consumption?	Often Results in What Effect on Weight?
Decreasing exercise		
No adult home after school		
TV watching		
Video games		
Computer use		

Critical Thinking

Childhood and adolescent obesity increase the likelihood of adult obesity. What is the potential socioeconomic impact of this trend on the future of healthcare?

_____

_____

_____

INVESTIGATION 6 What are the most common physiological changes that occur in older adults and how do these changes affect nutrient needs?

TEXT OUTLINE SUMMARY

16.5 Nutrition for young and middle adults, aged 19–64 years

    16.5.1 Adult growth and activity patterns

    16.5.2 What are an adult's nutrient needs?

    16.5.3 Nutrition-related concerns for adults

16.6 Nutrition for older adults, aged 65 years and older

    16.6.1 Older adult growth and activity patterns

    16.6.2 What are an older adult's nutrient needs?

        16.6.2.1 Energy and macronutrient recommendations for older adults

        16.6.2.2 Micronutrient recommendations for older adults

Study Questions

Answer these questions to develop the solution to the investigation.

What is one of the main reasons older adults are deficient in vitamin D? _____

Many retirees often fall into a very _____ lifestyle that has a negative impact on the physiological functions in their bodies.

Completion Exercise

Complete the following table indicating how each condition can be reversed and how nutritional changes can help.

Physiological Change	Can Be Positively Influenced by What?	Resultant Nutritional Change Needed
Decreased muscle mass	All can be positively influenced by significantly increased physical activity (exercise).	
Increased body fat		
Decreased bone density		
Decreased immune function		
Impaired nutrient absorption		

Critical Thinking

What role does a decreasing activity level in many older adults play with regard to nutritional needs?

_____

_____

_____

List the many benefits of older adults regularly engaging in a vigorous program of daily physical activity and exercise.

_____

_____

_____

INVESTIGATION 7   Why do many older adults avoid drinking adequate amounts of fluid?

TEXT OUTLINE SUMMARY

16.6.3   Fluid recommendations for older adults

16.6.4   Nutrition-related concerns for older adults

16.6.4.1   Overweight and underweight: a delicate balancing act

Study Questions

Answer these questions to develop the solution to the investigation.

Sensitivity to thirst often _____ with aging.

Urinary incontinence can _____ with aging.

Decreased fluid intake can lead to chronic _____ and hypernatremia (elevated blood sodium levels).

Critical Thinking

How do you think restroom availability in public spaces might contribute to insufficient fluid intake in older adults? Explain.

_____

_____

_____

INVESTIGATION 8   How can changes in dental health impact nutrient intake in older adults?

TEXT OUTLINE SUMMARY

16.6.4.2   Dental health issues

16.6.4.3   Other nutrition-related concerns

Study Questions

Answer these questions to develop the solution to the investigation.

Many older adults have serious dental problems that result in _____

chewing.

Lost teeth, gum disease, and/or poorly fitting dentures can cause people to avoid fresh

_____ and _____ and some _____.

Food avoidance can lead to severe _____ deficiencies in older adults.

Critical Thinking

What impact do you think socioeconomic status has on dental health and consequently on the overall health of older individuals? Explain.

_____

_____

_____

Answer Key

Chapter 1

INVESTIGATION 1

Terminology: See glossary.

Study Questions: nutrition; nutrition; nutrition

Completion Exercise: scurvy, mid-1700s, vitamin C, citrus fruits; pellagra, early 1900s, niacin, brewer's yeast

Critical Thinking: Answers will vary.

INVESTIGATION 2

Terminology: See glossary.

Study Questions: nutritional deficiencies; prevent deficiency diseases; chronic

Completion Exercise: See text Figure 1.1.

Critical Thinking: Answers will vary.

INVESTIGATION 3

Study Questions: health; disease

Completion Exercise: See Table 1.1 in text.

Critical Thinking: Answers will vary.

INVESTIGATION 4

Terminology: See glossary.

Study Questions: those that contain carbon; those that do not contain carbon

Critical Thinking: Answers will vary.

INVESTIGATION 5

Terminology: See glossary.

Study Questions: It does not support the regulation of body functions or the building and repairing of tissues; because they contain carbon and water; carbohydrates; fats; fats; proteins

Completion Exercise: Fats, 9, 90, 810, 32.4%; Proteins 4, 123, 492, 19.6%

Critical Thinking: Answers will vary.

INVESTIGATION 6

Terminology: See glossary.

Study Questions: Organic compounds that are required in small amounts and are necessary to regulate life processes; Vitamins are used for tissue growth and maintenance, immune system function and energy utilization; Fat-soluble vitamins include A, D, E, and K; Water-soluble vitamins include C and all of the Bs; Fat-soluble vitamins are stored in the body; Minerals are inorganic substances used by the body to promote normal function; Minerals are different from vitamins in that they do not contain carbon and are not changed or destroyed by heat or light; Major minerals need to be consumed in amounts greater than 100 mg/day, while trace minerals need to be consumed in amounts less than 100 mg/day.

Completion Exercise: Distinguishing features, see Tables 1.2 and 1.3; Foods − Fat-soluble = meats, dairy products, vegetable oils, avocados, nuts, and seeds; Water-soluble = grains, fruits, vegetables, meats, dairy products; Minerals (major and trace) = meats, dairy products, fruits, vegetables, and nuts

Critical Thinking: Answers will vary.

INVESTIGATION 7

Terminology: See glossary.

Study Questions: healthy; diseases; nutrient

Completion Exercise: See Figure 1.8.

Critical Thinking: Answers will vary.

INVESTIGATION 8

Study Questions: A registered dietician has a bachelor's degree, a licensed nutritionist is licensed by a particular state and may or may not have a degree in nutrition; A nutritionist is not an official title but simply someone who thinks they know something about nutrition; CDC; NIH

Completion Exercise: See Professional Organizations section in text.

Critical Thinking: Answers will vary.

Chapter 2

INVESTIGATION 1

Terminology: See glossary.

Study Questions: energy, nutrients, fiber; not eating too much or too little of certain foods; combinations of foods that provide the proper balance of nutrients; eating many different foods each day

Completion Exercise: Adequate: Eating enough of energy, nutrients, and fiber; Moderation: Not eating too much or too little of certain foods; Balance: Eating enough of foods from each group; Variety: Eating many different foods each day

Critical Thinking: Answers will vary.

INVESTIGATION 2

Terminology: See glossary.

Study Questions: nutritional facts panel; amounts of food typically consumed at a meal; 2,000; low; high

Completion Exercise: See text Figure 2.1.

Critical Thinking: Answers will vary.

INVESTIGATION 3

Terminology: See glossary.

Study Questions: U.S. Department of Agriculture and U.S Department of Health and Human Services; to help reduce the risk for chronic diseases; balance; 30; heart disease, type 2 diabetes, stroke, cancer

Completion Exercise: See Chapter 2 Nutrition Myth or Fact box: Alcohol can be a part of a healthful diet.

Critical Thinking: Answers will vary.

INVESTIGATION 4

Terminology: See glossary.

Study Questions: whole grains; variety; low-fat dairy; fish, nuts, vegetable oils; solid fats; 2–3 oz. or the size of a pack of playing cards; raw = 1 cup, cooked = ½ cup; your recommended calorie intake level

Critical Thinking: Will depend on personal dietary changes.

INVESTIGATION 5

Terminology: See glossary.

Study Questions: Following the MyPyramid will insure that you obtain enough energy, nutrients, and exercise to maintain health; MyPyramid recommends certain amounts of food groups to eat every day; by eating from each food group; include many colors of foods; smaller; developed the Healthy Eating Pyramid

Completion Exercise: See text Figure 2.5.

Critical Thinking: Answers will vary.

INVESTIGATION 6

Terminology: See glossary.

Study Questions: high fruit and vegetable consumption appears to decrease cancer and heart disease incidence; eat at least 5 servings of fruits and/or vegetables a day; to assess the effects of diet on hypertension; both stress the consumption of fruits and vegetables; heart disease and strokes would decrease

Critical Thinking: Answers will vary.

INVESTIGATION 7

Terminology: See glossary.

Study Questions: by the amount of carbohydrates, fat, protein, and calories in each food; starches/bread, meat, vegetables, fruits, milk, fat; fat, energy

Completion Exercise: See Table 2.7.

Critical Thinking: moderation

INVESTIGATION 8

Study Questions: about 4 times; high calories, high in fat, high in sodium

Critical Thinking: low fat, small portions (take some home), salads and low-fat dressings, less fried food, use appetizers for meal, etc.

Chapter 3

INVESTIGATION 1

Terminology: See glossary.

Study Questions: senses; appetite; hunger; holidays, events, location, time of day, watching TV, studying, stress

Critical Thinking: irritability and increase both; generally decrease

INVESTIGATION 2

Terminology: See glossary.

Study Questions: molecules; molecules

Completion Exercise: atoms; molecules; molecules; molecules

Critical Thinking: Answers will vary.

INVESTIGATION 3

Terminology: See glossary.

Study Questions: gatekeeper; two layers; phospholipid

Completion Exercise: See Figure 3.4 in text.

Critical Thinking: Answers will vary.

INVESTIGATION 4

Terminology: See glossary.

Study Questions: organs, digestive; mouth, esophagus, stomach, small intestine, large intestine, rectum; tongue, teeth, salivary glands, liver, gallbladder, pancreas

Completion Exercise: teeth, tongue, salivary glands, liver, gallbladder, pancreas; mouth, esophagus, stomach, small intestine, large intestine, rectum

INVESTIGATION 5

Terminology: See glossary.

Study Questions: mouth; propels food to stomach; mixes, digests, stores; small intestine; small intestine; large intestine

Completion Exercise: mouth—digestion; esophagus—none; stomach—digestion; small intestine—digestion, absorption; large intestine—elimination

Critical Thinking: Answers will vary.

INVESTIGATION 6

Terminology: See glossary.

Study Questions: -ase; mouth; salivary amylase; pepsin, gastric lipase; bile; pancreatic amylase, pancreatic lipase, proteases

Completion Exercise: breaks down starch; breaks down starch; breaks down proteins; breaks down proteins; breaks down fats; breaks down fats; breaks down starch; breaks down proteins; neutralizes stomach acid

Critical Thinking: Answers will vary.

INVESTIGATION 7

Terminology: See glossary.

Study Questions: esophagus; hydrochloric acid; not chewing food, eating late, overeating, alcohol; *Helicobacter pylori*; NSAIDS

Critical Thinking: Answers will vary.

INVESTIGATION 8

Terminology: See glossary.

Study Questions: diarrhea causes water loss that can quickly lead to dehydration; thirst, concentrated urine, dry skin; infrequent urination, crying without tears, fever, sunken abdomen, eyes, or cheeks, listlessness

Critical Thinking: Answers will vary.

Chapter 4

INVESTIGATION 1

Terminology: See glossary.

Study Questions: monosaccharides, disaccharides; sugars; glucose; monosaccharide; fructose; energy, sugar; polysaccharides; starch; glycogen; fiber

Completion Exercise: glucose; glucose; maltose; lactose

Critical Thinking: Answers will vary.

INVESTIGATION 2

Terminology: See glossary.

Study Questions: salivary amylase; disaccharides; small intestine; pancreatic amylase; maltase, sucrase, lactase; glucose; glycogen; fiber; insulin, glucagon

Completion Exercise: salivary amylase; pancreatic amylase; starch; sucrase; lactose; maltase

Critical Thinking: lack required enzymes; answers will vary

INVESTIGATION 3

Study Questions: energy; ketosis; protein

Critical Thinking: Answers will vary.

INVESTIGATION 4

Terminology: See glossary.

Study Questions: 130 grams; 45–65%

Critical Thinking: Answers will vary.

INVESTIGATION 5

Terminology: See glossary.

Study Questions: bacteria that cause tooth decay thrive on sugars; very little scientific evidence addresses this; increases LDLs; obese individuals tend to consume more dietary sugars than normal weight individuals

Critical Thinking: Answers will vary.

INVESTIGATION 6:

Study Questions: nondigestible carbohydrates; whole grains, fruits, vegetables; complex

Completion Exercise: Vegetables—corn 6, broccoli cooked 5, broccoli raw 3, collard greens 2; Fruits and Juices—blackberries 6, pear 5, apple 3, orange 3; Legumes—navy beans 8, kidney beans 8, black beans 7, lima beans 7; Breads and Cereals—oatmeal 4, whole-wheat bread 2, pumpernickel bread 2, bagel 2

Critical Thinking: Answers will vary.

INVESTIGATION 7

Terminology: See glossary.

Completion Exercise: none, 300; 15, 200; 50, 200; 5, 600

Critical Thinking: Answers will vary.

INVESTIGATION 8

Terminology: See glossary.

Study Questions: juvenile onset; inadequate insulin production; adult onset; insensitivity to insulin; too much insulin; lactase

Critical Thinking: Answers will vary.

Chapter 5

INVESTIGATION 1

Terminology: See glossary.

Study Questions: lipids; insoluble; triglycerides, phospholipids, sterols; triglycerides; fatty acids, backbone; fatty acids, backbone; sterols

Critical Thinking: Answers will vary.

INVESTIGATION 2

Terminology: See glossary.

Study Questions: carbon, hydrogen; hydrogen; double; one; tightly; adjacent; liquid; hydrogen, no; solid

Completion Exercise: None, Solid; One, Bent; Bent, Liquid

Critical Thinking: Answers will vary.

INVESTIGATION 3

Terminology: See glossary.

Study Questions: hydrogen atom, *cis;* liquid; *trans;* solid

Critical Thinking: Answers will vary.

INVESTIGATION 4

Terminology: See glossary.

Study Questions: small intestine; liver, gallbladder; when fat is present; breaks up fat molecules; chylomicron; phospholipid/protein surface layer; by the action of lipoprotein lipase

Completion Exercise: See Figure 5.6 in the main text.

Critical Thinking: Answers will vary.

INVESTIGATION 5

Terminology: See glossary.

Study Questions: twice the calories of carbohydrates and proteins; adrenaline promotes fat utilization; increases it; less; essential; fat, A, D, E, K

Completion Exercise: Vegetable oils, whole foods; Omega-3; regulation, heart protection

Critical Thinking: Answers will vary.

INVESTIGATION 6

Terminology: See glossary.

Study Questions: 20–30%; saturated and *trans;* less; approximately 10%, approximately 1%

Critical Thinking: Answers will vary.

INVESTIGATION 7

Terminology: See glossary.

Study Questions: hidden, saturated, *trans;* omega-3

Completion Exercise: 1st row—butter, safflower oil, chicken breast, olive oil, coconut oil; 2nd row—oils, walnuts, safflower oil, canola oil, palm oil; 3rd row—nuts, corn oil, walnuts, cashew nuts, 2% milk

Critical Thinking: Answers will vary.

INVESTIGATION 8

Terminology: See glossary.

Study Questions: phospholipids; HDL; VLDLs and chylomicrons; triglycerides and VLDLs; VLDL, LDL; HDL

Completion Exercise: 1st row—2%, 8%, 85%, 5%; 2nd row—10%, 18%, 52%, 20%; 3rd row—20%, 22%, 9%, 50%; 4th row—30%, 50%, 3%, 17%

Critical Thinking: Answers will vary.

Chapter 6

INVESTIGATION 1

Terminology: See glossary.

Study Questions: C, H, O; N; amino acids; synthesized; consumed; DNA

Completion Exercise: 1., 3., 5. = amine group; 2., 4., 6. = acid group; 7. = peptide bond; 8., 9. = amino acid; 10. = protein

Critical Thinking: Answers will vary.

INVESTIGATION 2

Terminology: See glossary.

Study Questions: complete; incomplete; complementary; mutual

Completion Exercise: Rice: incomplete, lysine, legumes; Beans: incomplete, methionine and cysteine, grains; Vegetables: incomplete, lysine methionine cysteine, legumes and grains *or* meat; Beef: complete, none, none

Critical Thinking: Answers will vary.

INVESTIGATION 3

Terminology: See glossary.

Study Questions: Crushed; broken into short polypeptides; broken into single amino acids; single amino acids, dipeptides, tripeptides; simple peptides; liver

Completion Exercise: Mouth: saliva, physical breakdown; Stomach: HCl, pepsin, protein broken into short polypeptides; Small intestine: proteases, short peptides into shorter peptides and single amino acids; Small intestine lining cells: none, all peptides broken down completely into single amino acids for absorption

Critical Thinking: Answers will vary.

INVESTIGATION 4

Terminology: See glossary.

Study Questions: Gastrointestinal lining; every 3–6 days; insulin; they pump Na^+ out of cells and K^+ into cells; buffers; to make antibodies to destroy the bacteria; when glycogen and fat stores are used up

Completion Exercise: 1. enzyme, 2. two separate compounds, 3. enzyme, 4. new compound on enzyme, 5. enzyme, 6. new compound

Critical Thinking: Answers will vary.

INVESTIGATION 5

Terminology: See glossary.

Study Question: 12–20%

Critical Thinking: Answers will vary.

INVESTIGATION 6

Terminology: See glossary.

Study Questions: Appears to go hand in hand; calcium; urea; urea

Critical Thinking: Answers will vary.

INVESTIGATION 7

Terminology: See glossary.

Study Questions: Meat, dairy; legumes; peas, garbanzo beans, kidney beans

Completion Exercise: Personal choices for this exercise

Critical Thinking: Answers will vary.

INVESTIGATION 8

Terminology: See glossary.

Study Questions: Marasmus; kwashiorkor, edema; protein-energy; DNA; PKU; abnormally; cystic fibrosis

Critical Thinking: Answers will vary.

Chapter 7

INVESTIGATION 1

Terminology: See glossary.

Study Questions: 50–70%; two-thirds; plasma, tissue fluid; electrolytes; sodium, potassium, chloride, phosphorus; as salts

Completion Exercise: Na, +, Na^+; K, +, K^+; Cl, −, Cl^-. P, −

Critical Thinking: Answers will vary.

INVESTIGATION 2

Terminology: See glossary.

Study Questions: amino acids, glucose, vitamins, minerals; fluid; low, hypotension; heat capacity; body; protection; lubrication

Critical Thinking: Answers will vary.

INVESTIGATION 3

Terminology: See glossary.

Study Questions: permeable, permeable; electrolytes; electrolytes; the membrane in the glass (like our cell membranes) is permeable to water and water moves from where there is more water (left side of the membrane) to where there is less water (the right side of the membrane where we find both water and salt). In other words, water follows electrolytes; the membrane in the glass (like our cell membranes) is not freely permeable to salt.

Critical Thinking: Answers will vary.

INVESTIGATION 4

Terminology: See glossary.

Study Questions: hypothalamus; sodium; drop; profuse sweating, blood loss, vomiting, diarrhea, low fluid intake; mouth

Critical Thinking: Answers will vary.

INVESTIGATION 5

Terminology: See glossary.

Study Questions: food and drink; carbohydrates; urine; sweating, breathing; feces

Completion Exercise: 300–400 ml, 1,000 ml, 1,200–2,350 ml; 1,400 ml, 900–2,150 ml, 200 ml

Critical Thinking: Answers will vary.

INVESTIGATION 6

Terminology: See glossary.

Study Questions: hypernatremia; hyponatremia; muscle cramps, loss of appetite, dizziness, fatigue, nausea, vomiting, mental confusion; increase salt consumption

Critical Thinking: Answers will vary.

INVESTIGATION 7

Terminology: See glossary.

Study Questions: dehydration; heavy, high; less body water, less efficient thirst mechanism responses; 1; thirst

Critical Thinking: Answers will vary.

INVESTIGATION 8

Terminology: See glossary.

Study Questions: high blood pressure; 25%, 50%; none; heart disease, stroke, kidney disease; 120/80

Completion Exercise: Decrease: salt consumption, smoking, alcohol consumption, weight; Increase: consumption of fruits and vegetables, low-fat proteins, and whole grains, exercise

Critical Thinking: Answers will vary.

Chapter 8

INVESTIGATION 1

Terminology: See glossary.

Study Questions: molecule; element; compound; oxidation; reduction; electron; free radical; electron; lipid

Completion Exercise: Normal oxygen; Oxygen with extra electron; Unpaired electron; Free radical

Critical Thinking: Answers will vary.

INVESTIGATION 2

Terminology: See glossary.

Study Questions: They become stable; vitamins, minerals, enzymes

Completion Exercise: Vitamins; Minerals (enzyme cofactors); Antioxidant enzymes, Beta-carotene; Phytochemicals

Critical Thinking: Answers will vary.

INVESTIGATION 3

Terminology: See glossary.

Study Questions: E; A; beta-carotene; C; selenium

Completion Exercise: E, vegetable oils; beta-carotene, red, orange, and yellow fruits and vegetables; A, animal foods; C, fresh fruits and vegetables; selenium, organ meats

Critical Thinking: Answers will vary.

INVESTIGATION 4

Terminology: See glossary.

Study Questions: enzyme activators; superoxide dismutase (SOD); copper, zinc, manganese; Catylase, iron; broken down into H_2O and O_2

Critical Thinking: Answers will vary.

INVESTIGATION 5

Study Questions: fresh fruits and vegetables; generally decreases them; organ meats; processed foods and junk foods

Critical Thinking: Answers will vary.

INVESTIGATION 6

Terminology: See glossary.

Study Questions: DNA damage; DNA; damaged; free radicals; antioxidant; antioxidant, decreased; immune

Critical Thinking: Answers will vary.

INVESTIGATION 7

Terminology: See glossary.

Study Questions: plants; lycopene, organosulfur compounds, flavinoids, phytoestrogens; cancer; increased; decrease

Completion Exercise: Answers will vary.

Critical Thinking: Answers will vary.

INVESTIGATION 8

Terminology: See glossary.

Study Questions: smoking, high blood pressure, high LDL, obesity, sedentary lifestyle; inflammation; prevent; antioxidants; E; fruits, vegetables, reduced

Critical Thinking: Answers will vary.

Chapter 9

INVESTIGATION 1

Terminology: See glossary.

Study Questions: 65, 35; strength, flexibility; structure; cortical, 80; trabecular, 20; trabecular

Completion Exercise: Cortical: 80, dense, outer surface of all bones and small bones, slow, more difficult; Trabecular: 20, light, ends of long bones and within flat bones, rapid, easier

Critical Thinking: Answers will vary.

INVESTIGATION 2

Terminology: See glossary.

Study Questions: Bone growth, bone modeling; Bone growth; Bone modeling; Bone remodeling; Increased, decreased; Increased, increased

Completion Exercise: Bone growth; Bone modeling; Bone remodeling

Critical Thinking: Answers will vary.

INVESTIGATION 3

Terminology: See glossary.

Study Questions: DEXA; dental; Postmenopausal women, risk factors; Peripheral; Wrist, heel

Completion Exercise: $-1 \rightarrow +1$: Normal bone density, comparable to a healthy 30-year-old; $-2.5 \rightarrow -1$: Low bone mass, increased risk for fractures; < -2.5: Osteoporosis

Critical Thinking: Answers will vary.

INVESTIGATION 4

Terminology: See glossary.

Study Questions: Calcium; Calcium; 2, 99; Acid-base balance, nerve impulse transmission, muscle contraction, maintenance of blood pressure, normal blood clotting, hormone regulation, and enzyme activation; Phosphorus, magnesium, fluoride; D, K

Completion Exercise: Vitamin D, sun, cod-liver oil; Vitamin K, vegetable oils, dark green leafy vegetables; Calcium, dairy products, dark green leafy vegetables; Phosphorus, meats, eggs; Magnesium, dark green leafy vegetables, whole grains; Fluoride, fluoridated water, fluoridated dental products

Critical Thinking: Answers will vary.

INVESTIGATION 5

Terminology: See glossary.

Study Questions: Dairy products; excellent; oxalates

Critical Thinking: Answers will vary.

INVESTIGATION 6

Terminology: See glossary.

Study Questions: Phosphoric acid; milk, calcium; calcium; caffeine

Critical Thinking: Answers will vary.

INVESTIGATION 7

Terminology: See glossary.

Study Questions: Due to increased bone fragility; Trabecular; Older adults

Critical Thinking: Answers will vary.

INVESTIGATION 8

Terminology: See glossary.

Study Questions: Less dense bones than males; Decreases; fruits, vegetables; calcium, D, exercise; Regular exercise; Decrease bone loss, increase bone density

Completion Exercise: Answers will vary.

Critical Thinking: Answers will vary.

Chapter 10

INVESTIGATION 1

Terminology: See glossary.

Study Questions: Enzymes are activated (become functional) when coenzymes are present; enzymes, coenzymes

Critical Thinking: Answers will vary.

INVESTIGATION 2

Terminology: See glossary.

Study Questions: coenzymes; increase

Completion Exercise: thiamine: carbohydrate, amino acid; riboflavin: carbohydrate, fat; niacin: carbohydrate, fat; pyridoxine: amino acid; folate (folic acid): amino acid; cobalamin: amino acid, fat; pantothenic acid: fat; biotin: carbohydrate, amino acid, fat

Critical Thinking: Answers will vary.

INVESTIGATION 3

Terminology: See glossary.

Study Questions: thiamine; riboflavin; pellagra; pregnancy; neural tube defects; pernicious

Completion Exercise: B_1: thiamine, beriberi; B_2: riboflavin, ariboflavinosis; B_2: niacin, pellagra; B_6: folic acid, neural tube defects; B_{12}: cobalamin; pernicious anemia

Critical Thinking: Answers will vary.

INVESTIGATION 4

Terminology: See glossary.

Study Questions: Carbohydrate, insulin; energy metabolism

Critical Thinking: Answers will vary.

INVESTIGATION 5

Terminology: See glossary.

Study Questions: Erythrocytes (red blood cells), leukocytes (white blood cells); Platelets; Leukocytes; Erythrocytes

Completion Exercise: plasma (liquid portion of the blood); leukocytes and platelets (buffy coat between the plasma and the red blood cells); erythrocytes (red blood cells)

Critical Thinking: Answers will vary.

INVESTIGATION 6

Terminology: See glossary.

Study Questions: Iron; Erythrocytes; Muscles; Oxygen transport; Vitamin C; Phytates; Increasing dietary iron intake; it can be fatal to small children if overconsumed; Women, menstruation

Critical Thinking: Answers will vary.

INVESTIGATION 7

Terminology: See glossary.

Study Questions: Folate, vitamin B_{12}; increases; increased; heart; brain; extremities

Critical Thinking: Answers will vary.

INVESTIGATION 8

Terminology: See glossary.

Study Questions: Without blood; Fatigue or lack of energy; Paleness

Completion Exercise: Iron deficiency: small, inadequate, iron; Pernicious; B_{12}; Macrocytic: large, inadequate, folate

Critical Thinking: Answers will vary.

Chapter 11

INVESTIGATION 1

Terminology: See glossary.

Study Questions: Look good, no need to diet, acceptable to you, promotes good eating habits and an active lifestyle; Obesity is overweight that is negatively affecting health

Completion Exercise: Too little body fat, looks skinny; Looks good; Too much body fat, body does not look proportionate; Excess body fat, general health is adversely affected; More than 100% overweight

Critical Thinking: Answers will vary.

INVESTIGATION 2

Terminology: See glossary.

Study Questions: Lean body mass, body fat; 18.5, 25; Diabetes, hypertension, heart disease; Skinfold method using a body fat caliper

Completion Exercise: Answers will vary.

Critical Thinking: Answers will vary.

INVESTIGATION 3

Terminology: See glossary.

Study Questions: Apple; energy expenditure; energy output, energy intake; energy intake, energy output; energy output, energy intake; Exercise; 60–70%

Completion Exercise: Decrease; Increase; Decrease; Increase; Don't change; Don't change; Increase; Decrease; Decrease; Increase; Don't change; Don't change; Increase; Decrease

Critical Thinking: Answers will vary.

INVESTIGATION 4

Terminology: See glossary.

Study Questions: Location has not been discovered yet; set point; Person tends to stay within a particular weight range and has minimal result from dietary changes; morbidly obese, lethargic, and die more quickly

Critical Thinking: Answers will vary.

INVESTIGATION 5

Terminology: See glossary.

Study Questions: Habits; couch potatoes or sedentary and heavy consumers of junk foods; Significant problem with obesity; medium to high parents and friends

Critical Thinking: Answers will vary.

INVESTIGATION 6

Terminology: See glossary.

Study Questions: Family and friends' pressure, expectations, food availability, TV, video games, computers, magazines with idealistic pictures; Increases it; Increases it; Cause them to develop an eating disorder so as to remain skinny

Critical Thinking: Answers will vary.

INVESTIGATION 7

Terminology: See glossary.

Study Questions: General overall lack of health and impaired disease resistance; Decreases lifespan and increases the risk of many diseases, including cardiovascular disease, diabetes, and joint problems; Cardiovascular disease, diabetes, hypertension

Completion Exercise: Answers will vary.

Critical Thinking: Answers will vary.

INVESTIGATION 8

Terminology: See glossary.

Study Questions: Energy intake, energy expenditure; The stomach can hold very little food so it is impossible to consume the volume of food that one had been able to consume prior to surgery; Decrease appetite or, by speeding you up, increase activity level

Completion Exercise: Answers will vary depending on personal opinions.

Critical Thinking: Answers will vary.

Chapter 12

INVESTIGATION 1

Terminology: See glossary.

Study Questions: Energy; not; subset; nutrition, physical activity; vigor, alertness

Completion Exercise: Answers will vary.

Critical Thinking: Answers will vary.

INVESTIGATION 2

Terminology: See glossary.

Study Questions: Heart disease, stroke, high blood pressure, obesity, type 2 diabetes, osteoporosis, colon cancer

Completion Exercise: sleep: improved; immune system: strengthened; anxiety: decreased; mental stress: decreased; depression: decreased; fatigue from chemotherapy: decreased; pregnancy and delivery: easier

Critical Thinking: Answers will vary.

INVESTIGATION 3

Terminology: See glossary.

Study Questions: Cardiorespiratory; Musculoskeletal; Muscular strength; Muscular endurance; Flexibility; body composition

Critical Thinking: Answers will vary.

INVESTIGATION 4

Terminology: See glossary.

Study Questions: Frequency, intensity, time

Completion Exercise: Answers will vary.

Critical Thinking: Answers will vary.

INVESTIGATION 5

Terminology: See glossary.

Study Questions: ATP; carbohydrates, fats, proteins; Glycolysis; pyruvic; lactic; lactic; fat (triglycerides); glucose; amino, repair

Critical Thinking: Answers will vary.

INVESTIGATION 6

Terminology: See glossary.

Study Questions: Carbohydrates; glycogen; moderate; repair; water; B-complex

Critical Thinking: Answers will vary.

INVESTIGATION 7

Terminology: See glossary.

Study Questions: Fluid, dehydration; heat syncope; heat cramps; heat exhaustion; heatstroke

Completion Exercise: Heat syncope: possibly, no, possibly; Heat cramps: yes, yes, possibly; Heat exhaustion: yes, no, excessive; Heatstroke: yes, no, none

Critical Thinking: Answers will vary.

INVESTIGATION 8

Terminology: See glossary.

Study Questions: Anabolic steroids; androstenedione, dehydroepiandrosterone; GHB; Creatine

Completion Exercise: Anabolic steroids: stunted growth, liver problems, cardiovascular problems, and reproductive problems; Testosterone precursors: can increase the risk of heart disease; GHB: seizures, death; Creatine: unknown

Critical Thinking: Answers will vary.

Chapter 13

INVESTIGATION 1

Terminology: See glossary.

Study Questions: Body image

Critical Thinking: Answers will vary.

INVESTIGATION 2

Terminology: See glossary.

Study Questions: Eating disorders; anorexia nervosa, bulimia nervosa; lower; abnormal, atypical

Critical Thinking: Answers will vary.

INVESTIGATION 3

Terminology: See glossary.

Study Questions: Family; unrealistic; sociocultural; anorexia; bulimia; genetic

Completion Exercise: Answers will vary.

Critical Thinking: Answers will vary.

INVESTIGATION 4

Terminology: See glossary.

Study Questions: Anorexia nervosa; anorexia; binge, purging; disorder; chronic

Completion Exercise: Anorexia nervosa: maintains body weight below normal; more common in females than in males; fear of weight gain, amenorrhea; severe nutrient deficiencies, then general organ/system dysfunction leading to death. Bulimia nervosa: binge eating followed by purging; more common in females than males, except in males who participate in "thin" male sports; episodic bingeing followed by compensatory behaviors aimed at preventing weight gain; gastrointestinal disturbances, electrolyte imbalances leading to death. Binge eating: stress leading to binge eating; very common in males, female-to-male ratio 1.5/1; obesity, low dietary restraint, low self-esteem; obesity-related health problems including heart disease, high blood pressure, stroke, diabetes, and arthritis, and psychological problems including social withdrawal and depression. Chronic dieting: restrained eater; similar in both men and women; preoccupations with food and weight, classifies foods as good or bad; can lead to a psychological eating disorder and altered BMR

Critical Thinking: Answers will vary.

INVESTIGATION 5

Terminology: See glossary.

Critical Thinking: Answers will vary.

INVESTIGATION 6

Terminology: See glossary.

Study Questions: Disordered eating, menstrual dysfunction, osteoporosis; estrogen, progesterone; leanness; less than

Critical Thinking: Answers will vary.

INVESTIGATION 7

Terminology: See glossary.

Study Questions: Team

Completion Exercise: Anorexia nervosa: nutritional counseling dealing with events and triggers; family therapy, group and individual counseling. Bulimia nervosa: restoring weight to normal range as soon as possible; family therapy, group and individual counseling

Critical Thinking: Answers will vary.

INVESTIGATION 8

Study Questions: Causes

Critical Thinking: Answers will vary.

Chapter 14

INVESTIGATION 1

Terminology: See glossary.

Study Questions: Seventy-six million; enzymes, microorganisms (bacteria); oxygen, heat, light

Completion Exercise: Answers will vary.

Critical Thinking: Answers will vary.

INVESTIGATION 2

Terminology: See glossary.

Study Questions: Microbes; microbes; food infections; food intoxications; neurotoxins; enterotoxins; allergies

Completion Exercise: *Campylobacter jejuni,* food poisoning; hepatitis A virus, hepatitis; BSE prion, mad cow disease; *Giardia lamblia,* giardiasis; molds, rarely cause food infections; *Clostridium botulinum,* botulism; *Aspergillus flavus,* affects multiple organs and can cause cancer and even death

Critical Thinking: Answers will vary.

INVESTIGATION 3

Terminology: See glossary.

Study Questions: Animal; greater; plant; cross contamination

Critical Thinking: Answers will vary.

INVESTIGATION 4

Terminology: See glossary.

Study Questions: Temperature; requirements

Completion Exercise: Sugaring: dehydration; Salting: dehydration; Drying: dehydration; Smoking: dehydration; Cooling: slows microbial growth; Canning: kills microbes in food; Pasteurizing: kills microbes in food; Chemical preservatives: prevent bacterial growth; Aseptic packaging: kills microbes in food and prevents bacterial growth; Irradiation: kills microbes; Genetic modification: can increase resistance to microbes

Critical Thinking: Answers will vary.

INVESTIGATION 5

Terminology: See glossary.

Study Questions: Ingredients; fats, oils; propionic acid; sulfites; to stop mold growth; nitrates and/or nitrites

Critical Thinking: Answers will vary.

INVESTIGATION 6

Terminology: See glossary.

Study Questions: FDA; taste, appearance, safety, nutrition; to replace flavor lost in processing; coal tar; tartrazine (FD&C yellow #5); measurable; cancer

Completion Exercise: flavorings: replace flavor lost in processing or enhance flavor; texturizers: improve texture; stabilizers: maintain smooth texture, uniform color and flavor; thickeners: thicken foods by absorbing some of the water; emulsifiers: stabilize oil-water mixtures; food colors: replace color lost in processing or enhance color; humectants: help to retain moisture in foods; desiccants: prevent foods from absorbing moisture from the air; vitamins: replace vitamins lost in processing or enhance nutrition; minerals: enhance nutrition; preservatives: extend shelf life

Critical Thinking: Answers will vary.

INVESTIGATION 7

Terminology: See glossary.

Study Questions: Crop; biopesticides; wash; EPA

Critical Thinking: Answers will vary.

INVESTIGATION 8

Terminology: See glossary.

Study Questions: Synthetic; USDA; 95; when all other natural measures fail

Critical Thinking: Answers will vary.

Chapter 15

INVESTIGATION 1

Terminology: See glossary.

Study Questions: Conception; folate; birth defects; abnormalities

INVESTIGATION 2

Terminology: See glossary.

Study Questions: Development, deficiencies; miscarriage, first; provide nutrients, remove fetal wastes; by the umbilical cord; premature, low birth weight

Completion Exercise: 1st: development of the nervous system and circulatory systems occurs, placenta and umbilical cord become fully developed and fully functional; 2nd: arms and legs are moving, bones and organ systems are developing, thumb-sucking starts, reactions to outside stimuli occur; 3rd: remarkable growth occurs (particularly of brain and lungs), hair appears

Critical Thinking: Answers will vary.

INVESTIGATION 3

Study Questions: 25–35 pounds; more, less.

Completion Exercise: 100 lbs: 128, 140; 150 lbs: 175, 185; 200 lbs: 215, 225; 250 lbs: less than 265, less than 265

Critical Thinking: Answers will vary.

INVESTIGATION 4

Terminology: See glossary.

Study Questions: Hormone; prolactin; oxytocin; stimulation; colostrum; it contains maternal antibodies

Critical Thinking: Answers will vary.

INVESTIGATION 5

Terminology: See glossary.

Study Questions: Increase; growth; nutrient; more

Completion Exercise: Energy: 700–800 kcal/day needed for milk production; Protein: to provide adequate protein for fetus/infant; Carbohydrate: to prevent ketosis; Folate: for normal neural tissue development; B_{12}: to prevent microcytic anemia; Calcium: to facilitate fetal/infant bone growth and to decrease maternal bone loss; Supplements: critical for brain growth and eye development; Fluid needs: to provide adequate amniotic fluid during pregnancy and to provide adequate fluid to produce milk during breast-feeding

Critical Thinking: Answers will vary.

INVESTIGATION 6

Terminology: See glossary.

Study Questions: Changes; infection, allergies; ovulation is suppressed; mother–infant bonding; economic

Completion Exercise: Answers will vary.

Critical Thinking: Answers will vary.

INVESTIGATION 7

Study Questions: High; eating, sleeping; triples; 50; intestinal cells do not make it yet; 2; 6–8

Completion Exercise: Fats: high energy yield, essential for normal nervous system growth and development; Proteins: difficult for infants to excrete excess amine groups from extra dietary protein intake; Carbohydrates: for energy

Critical Thinking: Answers will vary.

INVESTIGATION 8

Terminology: See glossary.

Study Questions: Introduce one new food at a time; vomiting and/or diarrhea; iron; nursing bottle syndrome; lead

Critical Thinking: Answers will vary.

Chapter 16

INVESTIGATION 1

Terminology: See glossary.

Study Questions: Increases; gradually slows; increases

Completion Exercise: Answers will vary.

Critical Thinking: Answers will vary.

INVESTIGATION 2

Terminology: See glossary.

Study Questions: Slightly; calcium, iron; 1: the beginning of sexual maturation; 2: in preparation for the adolescent growth spurt; menstruation begins

Critical Thinking: Answers will vary.

INVESTIGATION 3

Terminology: See glossary.

Study Questions: Heme; it is the most bioavailable; calcium; none

Completion Exercise: Iron: to prevent anemia; Protein: to facilitate growth, particularly muscle growth; Calcium: to facilitate normal skeletal development; Vitamin B_{12}: normal neurological development

Critical Thinking: Answers will vary.

INVESTIGATION 4

Terminology: See glossary.

Study Questions: Sexual; biologically; growth

Completion Exercise: Males: 4–12 inches; up to 45 pounds with a major increase in muscle mass and definition; lowering voice and appearance of pubic hair. Female: $2 \rightarrow 8$ inches; up to 35 pounds with body fat increase at buttocks, hips, thighs, upper arms and breasts; breast development, menarche, and pubic hair

Critical Thinking: Answers will vary.

INVESTIGATION 5

Study Questions: Too much, too little; less; less

Completion Exercise: All answers are "increased."

Critical Thinking: Answers will vary.

INVESTIGATION 6

Study Questions: Spend less time in the sun; sedentary

Completion Exercise: Decreased muscle mass: adequate protein intake; Increased body fat: decrease dietary fat; Decreased bone density: increase intake of vitamin D and calcium; Decreased immune function: increase intake of vitamins B_6 and B_{12}; Impaired nutrient absorption: increase intake of vitamins B_6 and B_{12}

Critical Thinking: Answers will vary.

INVESTIGATION 7

Study Questions: Decreases; increase; dehydration.

Critical Thinking: Answers will vary.

INVESTIGATION 8

Study Questions: Painful; fruits, vegetables, meats; nutrient

Critical Thinking: Answers will vary.